GUIDELINES
for Prescribing
FOOT ORTHOTICS

GUIDELINES
for Prescribing
FOOT ORTHOTICS

Mark A. Reiley, MD

Orthopedic Surgeon
Private Practice
Orthopedic Specialty Physician
University of California, Berkeley, Health Services
Berkeley, California

SLACK Incorporated, 6900 Grove Road, Thorofare, NJ 08086-9447

Publisher: John H. Bond
Acquisitions Editor: Amy E. Drummond
Associate Editor: Jennifer J. Cahill
Art Director: Linda Baker
Illustrations by D. Grant Ross

Reiley, Mark A.
Guidelines for prescribing foot orthotics/Mark A. Reiley; illustrations by D. Grant Ross.
p. cm.
Includes bibliographical references.
ISBN 1-55642-280-6 (alk. paper)
1. Orthopedic shoes. 2. Foot—Abnormalities—Treatment. 3. Leg—Abnormalities—Treatment. I. Title.
[DNLM: 1. Orthotic Devices—handbooks. 2. Foot Deformities—therapy—handbooks.
3. Foot Injuries—rehabilitation—handbooks. 4. Prescriptions, Non-Drug—handbooks. WE 39 R362g 1995]
RD757.S45R45 1995
617.5'8506—dc20
DNLM/DLC
for Library of Congress
95-17726

Printed in the United States of America
Published by: SLACK Incorporated
6900 Grove Road
Thorofare, NJ 08086-9447
Telephone 609-848-1000
Fax 609-853-5991
Contact SLACK Incorporated for further information about other books in this field or about the availability of our books from distributors outside the United States.

Last digit is print number: 10 9 8 7 6 5 4 3 2 1

CONTENTS

ACKNOWLEDGMENTS

The author would like to recognize and thank the following physicians who helped review, critique, and edit this manual.

Roger A. Mann, MD
    Clinical Professor of Orthopedics,
    University of California, San Francisco

Richard D. Ferkel, MD
    Foot and Ankle Surgeon,
    Orthopedic Institute,
    Van Nuys, California

Harry B. Skinner, MD
    Professor of Orthopedics,
    University of California, San Francisco

William Cimino, MD
    Foot and Ankle Surgeon,
    Private Practice,
    Oakland, California

Robert A. Eppley, MD
    Orthopedic Consultant,
    University of California, Berkeley

John McShane, MD
    Chief of Sports Medicine,
    University of California, Berkeley

ABOUT THE AUTHOR

Mark A. Reiley, MD, is an orthopedic surgeon in private practice in Berkeley, California. For 9 years he was on the clinical faculty of the University of California, San Francisco, during the first 3 years of which he worked at UCSF in the Musculoskeletal Tumor Clinic.

For the last 11 years, Dr. Reiley has been one of the Orthopedic Specialty Physicians for the University of California, Berkeley, Health Services, and has been the Chief Orthopedic Consultant for the Adult Hemophilia Clinic at Alta Bates Hospital in Berkeley.

At the present time, his professional interests are primarily the foot and ankle, musculoskeletal tumors, and joint replacement.

INTRODUCTION

The concept of computer-generated orthotics began in 1975. An inventor in Sunnyvale, California, went to a medical provider to have his foot pain evaluated. He was told he had flat feet and needed "orthotics." His feet were casted and then the casts were peeled off. He wondered if this primitive process would actually yield a product that would help his foot. Three weeks later, the hard plastic orthotics arrived and he attempted to wear them. The orthotics hurt his feet and never became comfortable even after several weeks. He thought a better system for orthotics could be invented. Over the next 10 years, he designed a computer system that could read a foot imprint and then use the image of that foot imprint to mill out an orthotic. Such a system would bypass the application and removal of casts. It also allowed the construction of an orthotic in the presence of the patient for immediate feedback.

In addition to his dislike of the existing orthotic making process, the inventor also believed that the hard plastic material chosen for the orthotic was too hard and not natural for the foot. As it happens, the medical literature supports the concept of wearing soft orthotics instead of hard plastic orthotics.

- Hard orthotics have been implicated in the etiology of several foot disorders, including sesamoiditis, neuromata, and stress fractures of the lower extremities.[1]

- Hard orthotics increase energy consumption in runners when compared to soft orthotics.[2]

- Soft orthotics cushion the foot more than hard orthotics, leading to less hematologic changes that can occur with running.[3,4]

- Soft orthotics allow some range of motion of the midtarsal joints which is important for proper load transfer across the foot.[5]

- Soft orthotics can extend for the length of the entire foot. Hard orthotics must end proximal to the metatarsal heads or they will break. This limits the effectiveness of hard orthotics especially in treating problems of the forefoot.

- Soft orthotics are cheaper and easier to adjust and/or replace than hard orthotics.

- Most orthopedic surgeons and sports medicine doctors believe rigid orthotics should be avoided whenever possible.[1]

The material eventually chosen for these computer-generated orthotics was ethyl vinyl-acetate (EVA). This material can be fabricated with durometric values from 20 to 75 durometers and still be "milled" by a metallic cutting ball into the shape desired. Orthotics made from EVA of less than 20 durometers do not hold up well. Orthotics of material 35 durometers do not control pronation or rearfoot motion well.[6] Orthotics made from EVA of 65 durometers are still flexible and yet are equal to hard plastic orthotics in decreasing the velocity of hindfoot pronation and in reducing the maximum angle of pronation of the foot.[7]

The system currently uses three densities of EVA depending on the type of orthotic required. If the patient has global foot problems such as diabetes mellitus, peripheral vascular disease, or rheumatoids with skin problems, then 30 durometer EVA orthotics are prescribed. All other orthotics are either 45 or 65 durometers, depending on two factors: if the orthotic is for a heavy individual or is only dress shoe length (two thirds the length of the foot), EVA of 65 durometers is used. Otherwise, EVA of 45 durometers is used.

As the developer of computer-generated orthotics experimented with his system, he noticed that orthotics made from a weight-bearing position of the foot seemed more comfortable than those made from a foot hanging off the edge of a table. The medical literature gives some support to imaging the foot in a weight-bearing position. In the first place, orthotics made from casts of a non–weight-bearing foot wind up being narrower than the foot when a person is standing.[8] Secondly, orthotics constructed from a foot in a non–weight-bearing position are shaped to a midfoot that is in excessive varus. In this position, the midtarsal joints are not able to move appropriately.[5,9] Midtarsal motion is essential to proper load disbursement in the foot.

He also noticed that external rotation of the tibia on a foot planted on the ground increases the medial longitudinal arch. He chose the position of the foot to be imprinted or "digitized" to be that position in which the Achilles is perpendicular to the ground and the foot is in a weight-bearing or partial weight-bearing position. This is identical to the neutral position described by Bordelon.[10]

Over the last 11 years, we have experimented with this orthotic system. During that time, I have prescribed just over 2000 orthotics. Of the first 600 prescriptions, approximately 100 of the patients were either not helped or helped only a little. During that time period, we only used the above described position, that of partial weight-bearing with the tibia rotated so that the Achilles was perpendicular to the ground, without modifications such as pads and wedges.

Since that initial period, we have learned how to utilize the orthotic modifications available in the computer. Modifications to heel height, hindfoot wedging, forefoot wedging, and padding are routinely added to the standard "neutral" position. The result is that now less than 3% of patients are dissatisfied with the inserts (as measured by guaranteed refunds for the orthotics).

The system for making computer-generated orthotics is a much more precise method of making and prescribing customized orthotics than any other currently used system. It is also the least expensive.

The following manual includes our current prescription recommendations for 32 painful foot and leg conditions. As the title of this books suggests these are guidelines for prescribing computer-generated foot orthotics. There is no perfect footprint or we would be able to prescribe inserts on the basis of a computer screen—which we cannot do.

In many cases, more than one thickness of heel height is suggested. In addition, although the computer can construct any degree of wedging, hindfoot wedging is prescribed as either a 5° or 9° wedge. The wedge is then rounded and shaped somewhat to a degree of wedging comfortable to the patient. As with all orthotics and prosthetics, the patient is the best source of feedback as to what is "correct." If further wedging of either the hindfoot or forefoot is needed, the orthotic can be easily modified at a later time.

PART ONE

PRINCIPLES ABOUT THE FOOT AND LEG RELEVANT TO ORTHOTICS

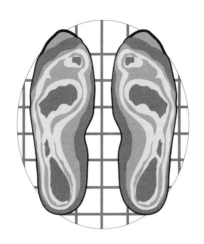

Foot Pronation
Cavus Foot
Leg Length Inequality
The "Q" Angle

FOOT PRONATION

[handwritten: • medical Hindfoot Wedge]

- All normal feet pronate with weight-bearing.

- Pronation is good for you since it helps absorb the impact of ground contact. It allows motion to occur at the midtarsal (talonavicular and calcaneocuboid) joints.[5,9]

[handwritten: ✱] • "Normal" pronation of the foot as measured by the navicular drop test is about 10 mm.[11] Nine to 11 mm is probably acceptable. Fifteen mm of navicular drop is clearly abnormal.[12,13]

- Overpronation increases the excursion of subtalar joint motion from 6° to 12°.[5] Over-excursion of the subtalar joint may cause increased stresses on the support structures of the medial longitudinal arch, including the plantar fascia, posterior tibialis, anterior tibialis, flexor digitorum longus, flexor hallucis longus, and spring ligament (Figure, page 10).[14]

[handwritten: ✱] • Five painful conditions commonly arise from hyperpronation. They are: plantar fasciitis, posterior tibial tendinitis, shin splints (anterior tibial myositis), patellofemoral arthralgia, and gluteus medius strain.[12,13]

[handwritten: ✱] • Other painful conditions that may arise from hyperpronation are less common but include: flexor digitorum longus tendinitis, flexor hallucis longus tendinitis, abductor hallucis myositis, posterior tibialis myositis, and iliotibial tract tendinitis.

[handwritten: • Stretch] • Tight heel cords work against or cause hyperpronation and need to be stretched.

[handwritten: • medical hind food wedge 5°] • Excessive pronation is treated with a medial hindfoot wedge. Start with a 5° medial wedge and increase to a 9° medial hindfoot wedge if needed.

CAVUS FOOT

[handwritten: • lateral hindfoot Wedge]

- Not a great foot.

- The weight-bearing area is decreased in a cavus foot.

- It is usually a stiff foot with very little subtalar motion and very little midtarsal motion during ambulation.

- Cavus feet can give rise to plantar fasciitis, iliotibial tract tendinitis, tarsal tunnel syndrome, metatarsalgia, and heel pain.

- Treat with a lateral hindfoot wedge. Start with a 5° wedge and advance to 9° of lateral hindfoot wedge.

- Also helped with Achilles stretching.

LEG LENGTH INEQUALITY

- Appears to cause little in the way of symptoms in the first two decades of life.[15]

- Beginning in the third decade, a short leg can cause problems with ipsilateral medial longitudinal arch support structures and the ipsilateral knee, due to an increased "Q" angle. The hip opposite the short leg can cause problems, usually in the form of trochanteric bursitis. In addition, leg shortness, even as little as one quarter of an inch, can cause mechanical low back pain.[12,13]

- In using a computer-generated orthotic to help correct a short leg syndrome, 3 mm to 9 mm can be comfortably added on to the short leg insert. Any further correction in leg length should be added to the outside of the shoe.

THE "Q" ANGLE

- The "Q" angle is the angle formed by a line connecting the anterior superior iliac spine, the patella, and the tibial tubercle.[16]

- An increased "Q" angle can result in anterior knee pain or retropatellar pain syndrome.[17] It can also aggravate iliotibial tendinitis.

- Decreasing the "Q" angle can decrease symptoms from retropatellar pain syndrome. It can also relieve some of the tension on the iliotibial tract.

- It is possible to decrease the "Q" angle by decreasing foot pronation. For every 1° increase in foot supination, there is a .44° decrease in the "Q" angle.[18] It is probably this relationship between foot pronation and the "Q" angle that accounts for the observation that 75% of runners' knee problems involve an abnormal foot.[9]

- Therefore, a 5° or 9° medial hindfoot wedge that increases foot supination can be used to treat either retropatellar pain syndrome or iliotibial tract tendinitis.

- Be advised that iliotibial tract tendinitis can be associated with a varus hindfoot, in which case, it is appropriately treated with a lateral hindfoot wedge.

PART TWO

THE ARCHES OF THE FOOT

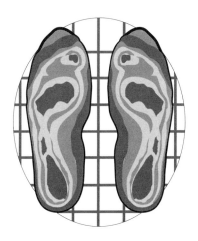

Relationships Between Arches
The Medial Longitudinal Arch
The Transverse Metatarsal Arch
The Lateral Longitudinal Arch

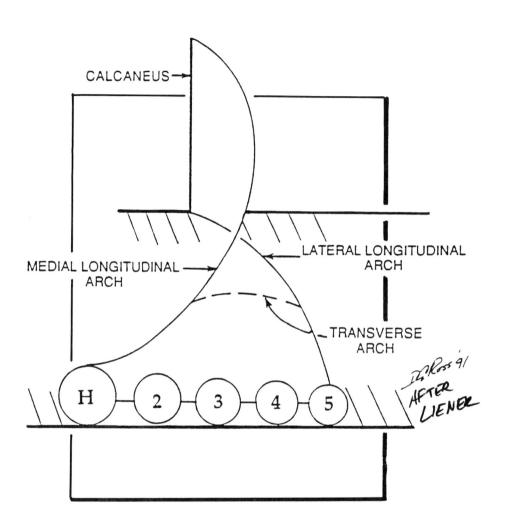

CALCANEUS

MEDIAL LONGITUDINAL
ARCH

LATERAL LONGITUDINAL
ARCH

TRANSVERSE
ARCH

H 2 3 4 5

RELATIONSHIPS BETWEEN ARCHES

There are three arches of the foot (Figure, page 8). The arches do not exist as separate entities. The transverse metatarsal arch is particularly sensitive to changes (ie, decreases) in the longitudinal arches. Rarely does one see the clinical consequences of a decreased transverse metatarsal arch (eg, metatarsalgia or interdigital neuroma) in a patient with a well-maintained medial longitudinal arch or a well-maintained lateral longitudinal arch.

The reason the transverse metatarsal arch height is related to the competence of the medial longitudinal arch and the lateral longitudinal arch is well illustrated in the Figure on page 12. This Figure (page 12) shows the peroneus longus as one of the supports of the transverse metatarsal arch of the foot. As is shown in the Figure on page 14, the peroneus longus is also one of the lateral longitudinal arch supports. Likewise, the Figure on page 12 also shows the posterior tibial tendon as a primary support for the transverse metatarsal arch, and the Figure on page 10 shows that tendon as a primary support for the medial longitudinal arch.

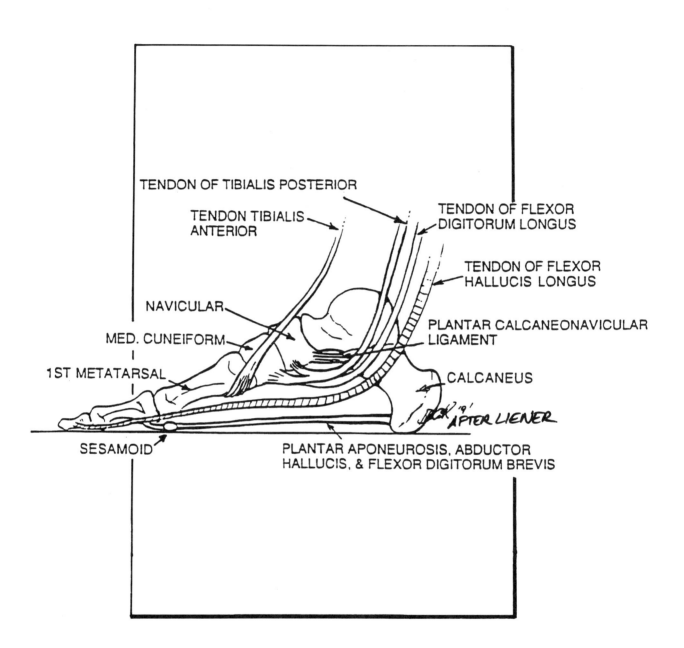

TENDON OF TIBIALIS POSTERIOR

TENDON TIBIALIS ANTERIOR

TENDON OF FLEXOR DIGITORUM LONGUS

TENDON OF FLEXOR HALLUCIS LONGUS

NAVICULAR

PLANTAR CALCANEONAVICULAR LIGAMENT

MED. CUNEIFORM

CALCANEUS

1ST METATARSAL

AFTER LIENER

SESAMOID

PLANTAR APONEUROSIS, ABDUCTOR HALLUCIS, & FLEXOR DIGITORUM BREVIS

THE MEDIAL LONGITUDINAL ARCH

According to Hamilton and Ziemer,[14] there are six main supports of the medial longitudinal arch (Figure, page 10). Those supports include: four tendons (anterior tibialis, posterior tibialis, flexor hallucis longus, and flexor digitorum longus) and two ligaments (the plantar "fascia" or aponeurosis and the "spring" or plantar calcaneonavicular ligament).

Any pathological condition that affects these structures will be improved by increasing the support of the medial longitudinal arch. One method already discussed is imaging the foot with the leg in external rotation to the point that the Achilles is perpendicular to the floor. All computer-generated orthotics start with this corrected position. Frequently, this amount of correction is not sufficient. Further support of the medial longitudinal arch must be added by prescribing either a medial forefoot wedge or a medial hindfoot wedge. If the uncorrected heel is in neutral position, then a medial forefoot wedge is prescribed. If the uncorrected hindfoot is in valgus, then a medial hindfoot wedge is prescribed.

In most patients, the medial longitudinal arch is corrected with a medial hindfoot wedge.

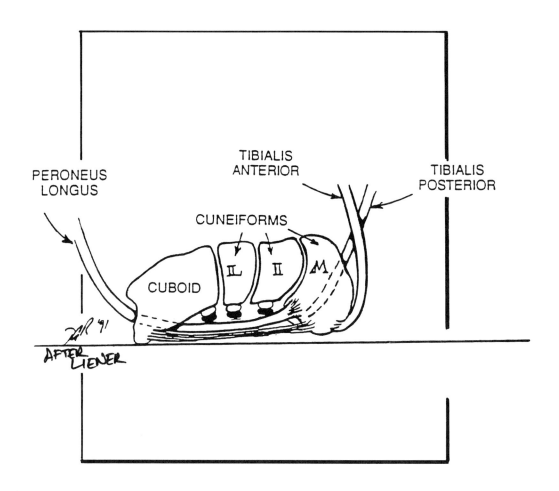

THE TRANSVERSE METATARSAL ARCH

The transverse metatarsal arch of the foot is illustrated in the Figure on page 12. This illustration diagrams the transverse metatarsal arch at the level of the cuneiform. The primary supports at this level include the peroneus longus (a lateral arch support) and the posterior tibial tendon (a medial arch support). In addition to the posterior tibial tendon, the long toe flexors, which also support the medial longitudinal arch, are shown under the cuneiform as supports for the transverse metatarsal arch of the foot. Laxity or injury to these structures affects not only longitudinal arch support but also support for the transverse metatarsal arch of the foot.

Transverse metatarsal arch problems, ie, forefoot problems, require a prescription that includes a forefoot pad somewhere and a wedge correction at one of the longitudinal arches of the foot.

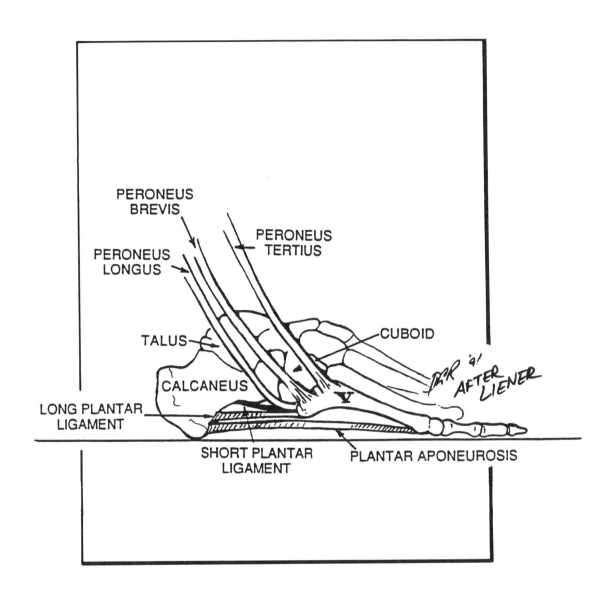

THE LATERAL LONGITUDINAL ARCH

The six primary supports of the lateral longitudinal arch of the foot are shown in the Figure on page 14. They include three tendons (peroneus longus, brevis, and tertius) and three ligaments (short plantar ligament, long plantar ligament, and plantar aponeurosis).

Painful conditions of these six structures are helped by increasing support of the lateral longitudinal arch. The support for the lateral longitudinal arch is increased with either a lateral hindfoot or a lateral forefoot wedge. If the uncorrected foot of the patient has a varus hindfoot when viewed from behind, then a lateral hindfoot wedge is prescribed. If a patient has a neutral hindfoot, then a lateral forefoot wedge is prescribed.

PART THREE

GAIT ANALYSIS AND ORTHOTIC PRESCRIPTION WRITING

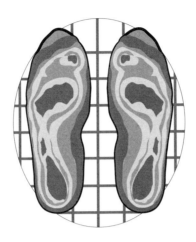

Gait Analysis and Foot Orthotics
Hindfoot Wedges
Neutral Heels
Forefoot Wedges
Heel Height
Forefoot Pads

GAIT ANALYSIS AND FOOT ORTHOTICS

- Gait analysis is a complex and intimidating topic. Volumes have been written about it and at least three formal systems for gait analysis have been described.[19]

- A complete formal gait analysis does not have to be done to prescribe computer-generated foot orthotics.

- For the purposes of foot orthotic prescription writing, gait analysis is only used to determine whether the hindfoot is in valgus, varus, or neutral position. This is determined by assessing the position of the medial malleolus during maximum single foot loading:

  If the medial malleolus moves toward the midline, the patient has a valgus hindfoot.

  If the medial malleolus does not move toward the midline and the Achilles tendon is perpendicular to the floor, the patient has a neutral hindfoot.

  If the calcaneus stays in varus position throughout weight-bearing, the patient has a varus hindfoot.

Please note the hindfoot includes the talus.

HINDFOOT WEDGES

Medial Hindfoot Wedges

When viewing the foot from the front, ie, with the patient walking toward the examiner, estimate the smallest distance between the floor and the medial longitudinal arch.

- If the distance is less than 3 mm, the patient is a severe pronator (regardless of how fast he or she resupinates). He or she will require either a 9° medial hindfoot wedge or a 5° medial forefoot wedge—at least to start. Remember that minor adjustments in the orthotics are immediately available to patients as they notice problems. It is easier to take away from an orthotic than to add to it. (Wedges greater than 9° are available, but most severe pronation problems respond to this degree of wedging.)

- If the distance is between 5 mm and 12 mm, the patient is a mild pronator and will require either a 5° medial hindfoot wedge or a 5° medial forefoot wedge.

- The decision to put the medial wedge in the forefoot or hindfoot is based on the position of the hindfoot. If the hindfoot when viewed from behind is in neutral, then a forefoot wedge is used. If the hindfoot is in valgus, then a hindfoot wedge is used. Again, remember the hindfoot includes the talus. A patient with a neutral appearing heel can still have a valgus hindfoot if the talar head pronates. (See discussion on Neutral Heels.)

- If the distance is greater than 15 mm, the patient needs to be viewed from the back to see if the hindfoot is in varus or valgus at maximum single foot loading. In addition, make sure that the patient is walking "unconsciously." Have the patient think about grocery shopping while walking. Also, if the patient has an antalgic (painful) limp, ask him to try to walk normally and ignore the pain. Otherwise, orthotic gait analysis is useless.

Lateral Hindfoot Wedges

Lateral hindfoot wedges account for only 5% to 10% of our orthotic prescriptions. When viewing the foot from the back, ie, with the patient walking away from the examiner, the position of the hindfoot should be checked with relation to the neutral position.

- If the hindfoot remains in 5° of varus or more during maximum single foot loading, then a 9° lateral hindfoot wedge is prescribed.

- If the hindfoot reaches 1° to 4° of varus during maximum loading, then a 5° lateral hindfoot wedge is prescribed.

- If the hindfoot is in neutral position, then wedging is performed in the forefoot.

- If the hindfoot reaches a valgus position, then a medial wedge is needed.

NEUTRAL HEELS

If a patient has a neutral hindfoot, ie, a hindfoot which when viewed from behind is in neither varus nor valgus, then a neutral heel is prescribed. All wedging of a foot with a neutral hindfoot is done in the forefoot.

The assessment of a neutral hindfoot is not straightforward. When examining a patient's gait from behind, it can occasionally appear as if the calcaneus and Achilles remain perpendicular to the floor. Thus, this would seem to be a neutral hindfoot. However, this may not be the case because the hindfoot also includes the talus, and not infrequently the calcaneus appears to be neutral, but the head of the talus can still sag into a valgus position in the full weight-bearing single leg stance position. In such a patient, the hindfoot would be assessed as valgus even though the heel is in neutral, and the patient would be prescribed a medial hindfoot wedge instead of a forefoot wedge.

FOREFOOT WEDGES

A medial forefoot wedge is prescribed for a patient with a neutral or varus hindfoot and a medial forefoot problem.

Lateral forefoot wedges are more commonly prescribed. A lateral forefoot wedge is combined with either a medial hindfoot wedge or a neutral heel in order to increase medial-lateral stability. Currently, the diagnoses treated with a lateral forefoot wedge include:

- Metatarsalgia of the 4th and 5th metatarsal heads

- Neuroma between the 4th and 5th metatarsal heads

- Dorsal subluxation of the base of the 4th metatarsocuboid joint with a valgus hindfoot

- Stress fractures of the 4th and 5th metatarsal shafts

- Plantar fasciitis with a neutral hindfoot and a hypermobile 1st ray

HEEL HEIGHT

The heel height of the wedges can be altered from 0 mm to 9 mm. Beyond 9 mm, the heel tends to lift out of the average shoe.

The following conditions all require low (1 mm) heel height:

- All forefoot problems

- All midfoot problems

- All dysvascular and neuropathic feet, unless a sore on the heel is present

- Shin splints (anterior tibial myositis)

- Anterior tibial tendinitis

- Lateral ankle instability

- All knee conditions listed in this handbook

- Osteochondritis dissecans of the posteromedial talar dome

- Plantar fasciitis (unless the Achilles tendon is too tight)

For the following conditions, a 3 mm heel is recommended:

- Osteochondritis dissecans of the anteromedial talar dome

- Lateral ankle impingement

- Tarsal tunnel syndrome

- Short leg

- Posterior tibial tendinitis (see also 9 mm heel height)

- Flexor digitorum longus and flexor hallucis longus tendinitis (see also 9 mm heel height)

A 9 mm heel height is recommended for the following conditions:

- Achilles tendinitis

- Post-Achilles repair

- Calcaneal apophysitis

- Early treatment of posterior tibial tendinitis, flexor hallucis longus tendinitis, flexor digitorum longus tendinitis

- Plantar fasciitis (if the gastroc-soleus complex is exceedingly tight)

FOREFOOT PADS

The forefoot is everything distal to the metatarsal bases.[20]

- Forefoot problems are worsened by hyperpronation or cavus deformities, and thus it is useful to correct hindfoot position problems with a medial or lateral hindfoot wedge (see above), rather than just giving a patient a metatarsal pad.

- All forefoot conditions and dorsal subluxations of the base of the 4th metatarsal require prescription of a forefoot pad.

- All forefoot conditions are helped by reducing heel height and by encouraging daily calf stretching. Please note that stretching the calf for less than 30 seconds actually winds up tightening the calf muscles.

PART FOUR

STRETCHING

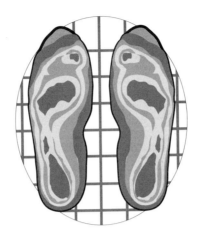

The Gastrocnemius Stretch

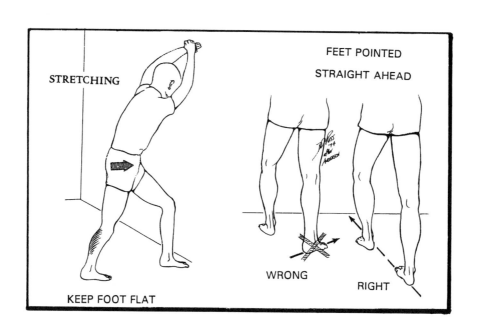

STRETCHING

KEEP FOOT FLAT

FEET POINTED STRAIGHT AHEAD

WRONG

RIGHT

THE GASTROCNEMIUS STRETCH

- For many if not all of the conditions in this manual, calf stretching is one of the cornerstones of treatment.

- Mann asserts that wedged heels, arch supports, or heel cups are ineffective in the face of a tight heel cord unless the calf is assiduously stretched.[5]

- Patients need to be taught repeatedly how to stretch. All patients in my practice who are taught how to stretch are followed up in 1 month to check their progress. At that visit, they are asked to demonstrate proper calf stretching technique. One hundred percent of patients demonstrate improper technique and have to be retaught. Even when patients are told beforehand that they will be asked to demonstrate proper stretching, 100% will still not stretch their calves correctly.

- Calf stretching, if done for less than 30 seconds, actually tightens the calf muscle, making the problem being treated worse.[21-23]

- Only the muscle stretches, not the tendon. If a person feels the stretch in the heel or in the Achilles tendon, he or she is pushing too hard.

- Calf stretching should be done with the toes pointing toward the wall and not externally rotated (Figure, page 26). Otherwise, the foot bends at the talonavicular and calcaneocuboid joints and the calf muscle is not stretched. Also, it is best if the patient wears his or her orthotic while stretching.

- Calf stretching should be performed five times per day.

PART FIVE

SHOES AND ORTHOTICS

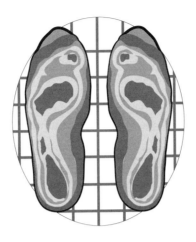

Athletic Shoes and Orthotics
Shoes for Men
Shoes for Women

ATHLETIC SHOES AND ORTHOTICS

- The importance of shoewear cannot be overemphasized.

- Shoe type has been shown to influence oxygen consumption in both walking and running.[24,25] This influence on oxygen consumption is due to geometric factors and differences in shock absorption, not to weight differences.[26-29]

- A sturdy, well-fitted rigid heel counter has been found to decrease both oxygen consumption and muscle load in the triceps surae,[30] thereby reducing the potential for overuse injuries. Most of the conditions described in this manual are overuse syndromes.

- The computer-generated orthotic—or any orthotic for that matter—is only as good as the shoe it is sitting in. Any orthotic in a $19 pair of canvas boat shoes is going to be ineffective.

- Current recommendations for shoewear for men and women are listed on the following two pages (Tables 1 and 2). Please note that these tables were compiled in 1995 and will no doubt be obsolete by 1996 due to the ever changing shoe industry.

	TABLE 1	
	Shoes for Men	
Patient Problem	**Need**	**Recommended Shoe**
Weight Hard on shoes	Rigid sole Stability Durability	New Balance: 997, 577, 906, 806, 540 Asics: Gel MC, GT Intensity K-Swiss: Gstaad Avia: 2050
Pronation Flat feet	Semi-curved or straight last Medial support Firm heel counter	Asics: Gel MC, 2001 Saucony: Vang New Balance: 998, 580 Avia: 2052
Supination	Curved last Lateral support Firm heel counter Soft, neutral mid sole	Saucony: Shadow 6000, G.R.I.D. Shadow New Balance: 906, 806, 997, 540, CXT 770, 577 Wilson: Plexus Asics: GT Intensity
Flexibility	Rigid sole	New Balance: 650 Avia: 2052 Asics: V-2 Wilson: Pro Staff Reebok: Satellite Low
Weak ankle	Ankle support	Avia: 2052 Saucony: Vang
Bunion Wide forefoot Neuroma	Firm heel counter Wide forefoot	Saucony: G.R.I.D. Shadow, Vang, 6000 Avia: 2052 New Balance: in widths
Heel spur Plantar fasciitis	Firm heel counter Cushioning	New Balance: 998, CT 320 Saucony: all Asics: 2001 Avia: 2052
Narrow feet	Narrow shoe	New Balance: in narrow widths Avia: 2050 Saucony: G.R.I.D. Shadow

TABLE 2
Shoes for Women

Patient Problem	Need	Recommended Shoe
Weight Hard on shoes	Rigid sole Stability Durability	New Balance: 997, 526, 506 Avia: 351, 2050, 1387 Asics: GT Intensity Wilson: Pro Staff, Plexus
Pronation Flat feet	Semi-curved or straight last Medial support Firm heel counter	Asics: 2001 Saucony: Vang New Balance: 998, 680 Avia: 2052
Supination	Curved last Lateral support Firm heel counter Soft, neutral mid sole	Saucony: Shadow 6000, Jazz 5000, G.R.I.D. Shadow New Balance: 998 Wilson: Plexus Asics: GT Intensity Avia: 455, 450
Flexibility	Rigid sole	Saucony: Vang Avia: 1470 Asics: Gel-Catalyst Wilson: Pro Staff Reebok: Satellite Low
Weak ankle	Ankle support	Avia: 2052 Saucony: Vang
Bunion Wide forefoot Neuroma	Firm heel counter Wide forefoot	Saucony: Shadow 6000, Vang, G.R.I.D. Shadow Avia: 2052 New Balance: in widths
Heel spur Plantar fasciitis	Firm heel counter Cushioning	New Balance: 998, CT 300 Saucony: all Asics: 2001 Avia: 2052
Narrow feet	Narrow shoe	New Balance: in narrow widths Saucony: G.R.I.D. Shadow

PART SIX
FOREFOOT CONDITIONS

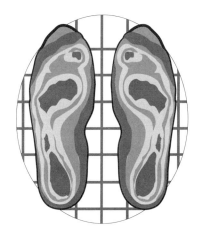

Hammer Toes
Morton's Neuroma
Metatarsalgia (1st, 2nd, and 3rd metatarsal heads)
Metatarsalgia (4th and 5th metatarsal heads)
Sesamoiditis
Turf Toe (hyperextension type)
Hallux Rigidus
Hallux Valgus
Metatarsal Stress Fractures

AREAS OF TENDERNESS

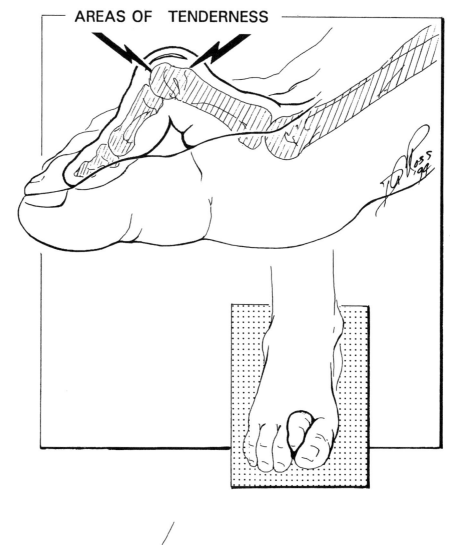

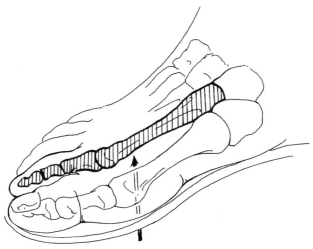

PAD PROXIMAL TO INVOLVED TOE

36

HAMMER TOES

- A hammer toe is a flexion deformity of the PIP joint of the lesser toes.

- A claw toe is a hammer toe with an associated extension deformity of the metatarsal phalangeal joint.

- In years past, hammer toes and claw toes were felt to be due to imbalance in the intrinsics of the foot; however, this has not been experimentally demonstrated in several attempts.[31] When patients have a flexible hammer toe, they are often helped with anterior tibial strengthening done with the foot held in a supinated position. This observation leads one to theorize that these conditions are the result of an extrinsic imbalance.

- Hammer toes of the 2nd and 3rd toes are improved with a slight increase in the medial longitudinal arch by using either a medial hindfoot or medial forefoot wedge and support of the transverse metatarsal arch with a metatarsal pad.

- Hammer toes of the 4th and 5th toes are improved by increasing the lateral longitudinal arch by using a lateral hindfoot or lateral forefoot wedge and a metatarsal pad to support the transverse metatarsal arch.

- As with all forefoot conditions, a tight Achilles tendon is most likely present and thus a low (1 mm) heel is needed.

- Hammer toe deformities of all four lesser toes are helped by wearing a shoe with a large toe box.

Hammer Toes of the 2nd and 3rd Rays

If the hindfoot is in valgus:

- Rx: 5° or 9° medial hindfoot wedge
    Pad proximal to involved toe
    1 mm heel height

If the hindfoot is in neutral:

- Rx: 0° hindfoot wedge plus 5° medial forefoot wedge
    Pad proximal to involved toe
    1 mm heel height

Hammer Toes of the 4th and 5th Rays

If the hindfoot is in neutral:

- Rx: 0° hindfoot wedge plus 5° lateral forefoot wedge
    Pad proximal to involved toe
    1 mm heel height

If the hindfoot is in varus:

- Rx: 5° lateral hindfoot wedge
    Pad proximal to involved toe
    1 mm heel height

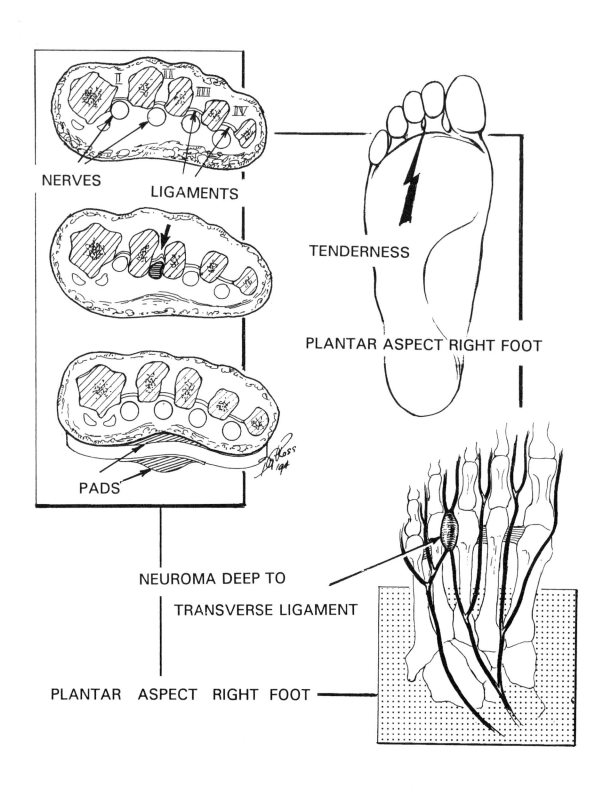

NERVES

LIGAMENTS

TENDERNESS

PLANTAR ASPECT RIGHT FOOT

PADS

NEUROMA DEEP TO

TRANSVERSE LIGAMENT

PLANTAR ASPECT RIGHT FOOT

MORTON'S NEUROMA

- Compression of the common digital nerve located between the metatarsal heads.

- Tenderness is found between the metatarsal heads, not on the heads.

- One theory on the cause of Morton's neuromas suggests that the interdigital nerve is irritated by the intermetatarsal ligament which sags plantarward toward the nerve as the height of the transverse metatarsal arch decreases.

- Treat with a metatarsal pad proximal to the involved interspace. This pad helps elevate the transverse metatarsal arch at the area of the neuroma.

- Correction of the longitudinal arches is also prescribed depending on which is deficient.

- Shoes with wide toe boxes should be worn, and high heeled shoes should be avoided.

Neuroma Medial to 4th Metatarsal

If the hindfoot is in valgus:

- Rx: 5° or 9° medial hindfoot wedge
    Pad proximal to 2nd or 3rd metatarsal head
    1 mm heel height

If the hindfoot is in neutral:

- Rx: 0° medial forefoot wedge and 5° medial forefoot wedge
    Pad proximal to 2nd or 3rd metatarsal head
    1 mm heel height

Neuroma between the 4th and 5th Metatarsal Heads*

If the hindfoot is in neutral:

- Rx: 0° medial hindfoot wedge and 5° lateral forefoot wedge
    Pad proximal to 4th metatarsal head
    1 mm heel height

If the hindfoot is in varus:

- Rx: 5° lateral hindfoot wedge
    Pad proximal to 4th metatarsal head
    1 mm heel height

*Many foot and ankle surgeons do not believe neuromas occur in the interspace of the 4th and 5th metatarsal heads (Mann, personal communication, 1993).

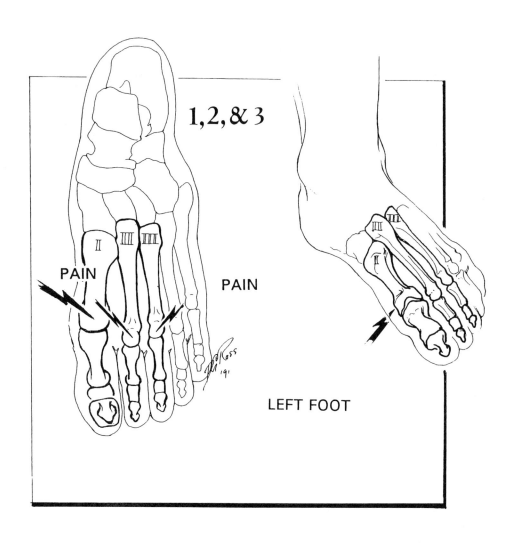

1, 2, & 3

PAIN

PAIN

LEFT FOOT

METATARSALGIA
(1ST, 2ND, AND 3RD METATARSAL HEADS)

- Metatarsalgia of the 1st or great metatarsal head is sesamoiditis (page 44).

- Weight-bearing of the forefoot is supposed to be evenly distributed between six structures: the two sesamoids under the 1st head and the four heads of the lesser metatarsals.

- Metatarsalgia occurs when forefoot weight-bearing is maldistributed.

- Metatarsalgia of the 2nd and 3rd heads is treated with a medial hindfoot wedge and a pad just proximal to the involved head.

- The condition is also helped with daily calf stretching and toe grasping exercises.

If the hindfoot is in valgus:

- Rx: 5° or 9° medial hindfoot wedge
    Pad proximal to the 2nd or 3rd metatarsal head
    1 mm heel height*

    If the hindfoot is in neutral:

- Rx: 0° hindfoot wedge
    5° medial forefoot wedge
    Pad proximal to 2nd or 3rd metatarsal head
    1 mm heel height*

*Early stages of avascular necrosis of the 2nd metatarsal head (Frieberg's infraction) or of the 3rd metatarsal head may also be symptomatically improved with this orthotic prescription.[32]

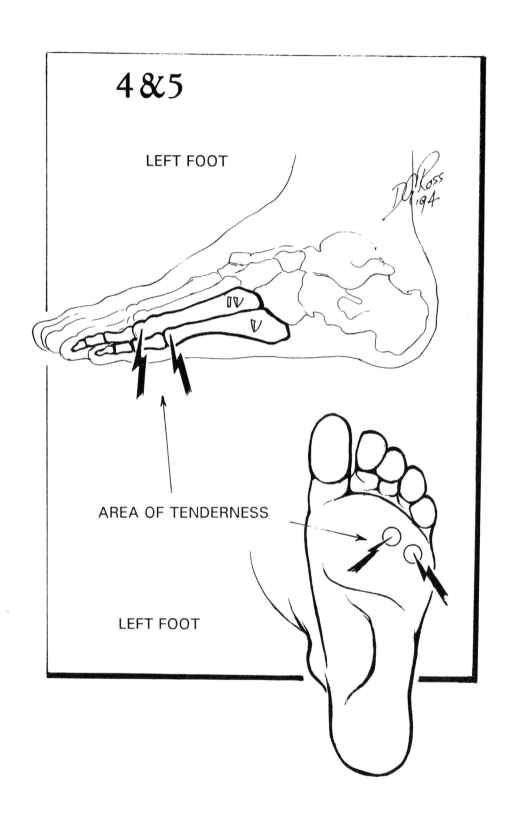

4 & 5

LEFT FOOT

AREA OF TENDERNESS

LEFT FOOT

METATARSALGIA
(4TH AND 5TH METATARSAL HEADS)

- See discussion in previous section on page 41.

- As in all forefoot problems, calf stretching is the cornerstone of conservative management.

- Treatment of metatarsalgia of the 4th or 5th metatarsal heads varies depending on the amount of hindfoot varus.

If the hindfoot is in neutral:

- Rx: 0° hindfoot wedge
     5° lateral forefoot wedge
     Pad just proximal to the 4th and 5th heads
     1 mm heel height

If the hindfoot is in varus:

- Rx: 5° hindfoot wedge
     Pad just proximal to the 4th and 5th heads
     1 mm heel height

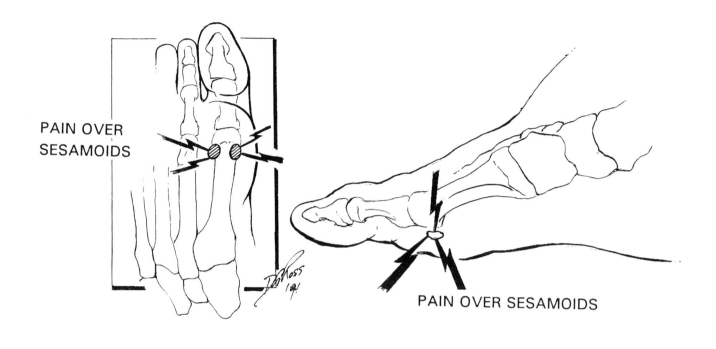

PAIN OVER
SESAMOIDS

PAIN OVER SESAMOIDS

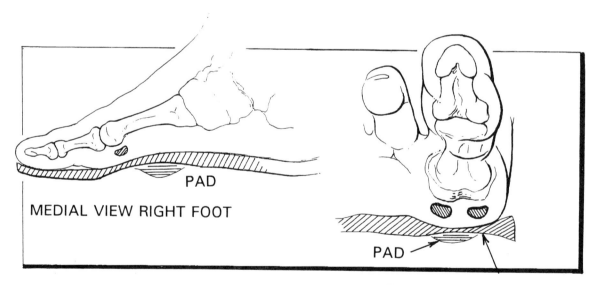

MEDIAL VIEW RIGHT FOOT

PAD

PAD

ROUTED OUT FOR SESAMOIDS

SESAMOIDITIS

- Two sesamoids are situated under the great metatarsal head.

- Each sesamoid bears one sixth of the forefoot weight.

- This condition is diagnosed by tenderness over either sesamoid.

- Treat with a medial longitudinal arch correction and a pad just proximal to the sesamoids.

- It is sometimes helpful to grind or rout away a portion of the insert beneath the sesamoids.

- As in all forefoot problems, slow, gentle calf stretching several times a day is indicated.

- Avoid high heeled shoes.

If the hindfoot is in valgus:

- Rx: 5° or 9° medial hindfoot wedge and pad just proximal to the sesamoids
    Grind out area under sesamoids
    1 mm heel height

If the hindfoot is in neutral:

- Rx: 0° hindfoot wedge
    5° medial forefoot wedge and pad proximal to the sesamoids
    Grind out area under sesamoids
    1 mm heel height

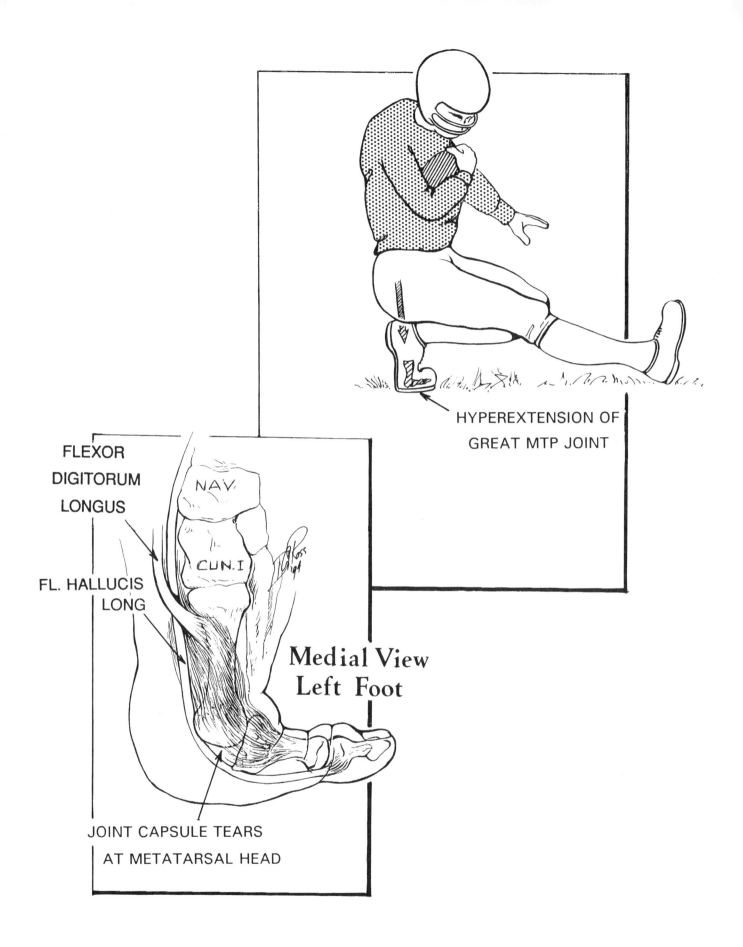

HYPEREXTENSION OF
GREAT MTP JOINT

FLEXOR
DIGITORUM
LONGUS

NAV.

CUN. I

FL. HALLUCIS
LONG

Medial View
Left Foot

JOINT CAPSULE TEARS
AT METATARSAL HEAD

TURF TOE
(HYPEREXTENSION TYPE)

- A turf toe is the name given to a traumatic injury of the great metatarsal phalangeal joint. Usually it occurs in an athlete wearing flexible shoes. Frequently, but not always, it occurs on artificial turf.[33]

- The injury can be caused by hyperextension, hyperflexion, or collateral ligament trauma. The type of injury is diagnosed by history and by palpation of the foot.

- Turf toe patients may have decreased range of motion of the great metatarsal phalangeal joint for 1 year following injury. This type of injury may be a precursor to hallux rigidus.

- During the period of acute pain, the patient may be helped by spica taping of the great toe for short periods.

- A hyperextension turf toe should be treated by an orthotic device and shoe combination that prevents extension of the great metatarsal joint.

- A hyperextension type turf toe is worsened with pronation.[33]

If the hindfoot is in valgus:

- Rx: 5° or 9° medial hindfoot wedge
  Pad proximal to great metatarsal phalangeal joint
  Stiff soled shoe (rocker soled shoe may also help)
  1 mm heel height

If the hindfoot is in neutral:

- Rx: 0° hindfoot wedge
  5° lateral forefoot wedge
  Pad proximal to great metatarsal phalangeal joint
  Stiff soled shoe
  1 mm heel height

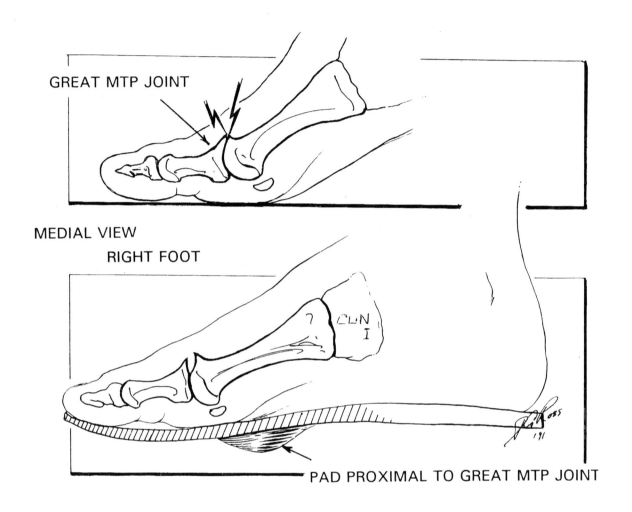

GREAT MTP JOINT

MEDIAL VIEW

RIGHT FOOT

PAD PROXIMAL TO GREAT MTP JOINT

48

HALLUX RIGIDUS

- Hallux rigidus is a condition that causes pain at the great metatarsal phalangeal joint due to arthritis and spurring.

- Pain is found on the dorsum of the great MTP joint, especially with extension.

- Treat by limiting extension of the great MTP joint, which is done by placing a pad proximal to the MTP joint. In addition, it helps to increase the weight-bearing of the lateral foot with a medial hindfoot wedge.

- Appropriate calf stretching is indicated, as in all forefoot problems.

If hindfoot is in valgus:

- Rx: 5° or 9° medial hindfoot wedge and pad just proximal to the great metatarsal phalangeal joint
    Stiff soled shoe
    1 mm heel height

If hindfoot is in neutral:

- Rx: 0° hindfoot wedge
    5° medial forefoot wedge and pad proximal to the great metatarsal phalangeal joint
    Stiff soled shoe
    1 mm heel height

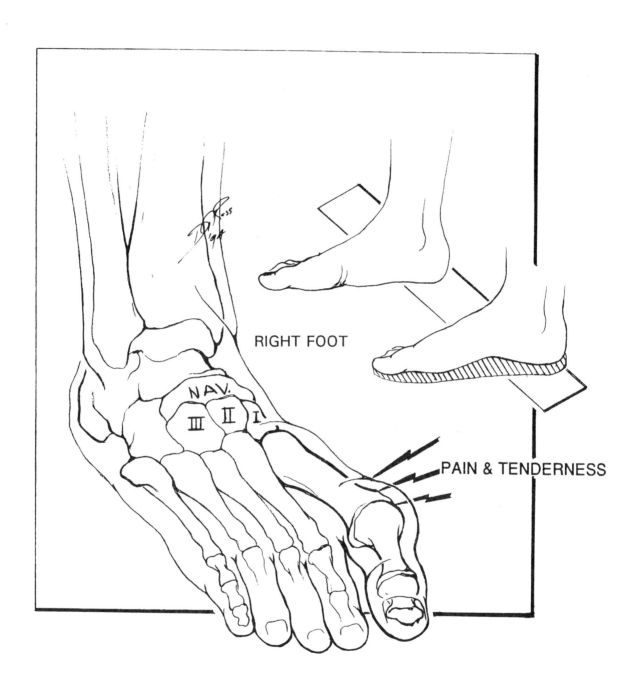

RIGHT FOOT

NAV.

III II I

PAIN & TENDERNESS

HALLUX VALGUS

- Hallux valgus includes several foot deformities:
    - A decrease in the medial longitudinal arch
    - A medially deviated great metatarsal
    - A laterally deviated great toe (hallux valgus)

- Pain is on the medial side of the MTP joint, not on the top or the bottom.

- The role of pronation of the foot in the pathophysiology of hallux valgus has been clearly delineated.[5]

- If a hammer toe is present, add a metatarsal pad.

- Appropriate calf stretching is indicated as in all forefoot problems.

If the hindfoot is in valgus:

- Rx: 5° or 9° medial hindfoot wedge*
    - Add metatarsal pads if metatarsalgia is present
    - 1 mm heel height
    - Shoe with wide toe box

If the hindfoot is in neutral:

- Rx: 0° hindfoot wedge
    - 5° medial forefoot wedge
    - 1 mm heel height
    - Metatarsal pad as needed
    - Shoe with wide toe box

*These inserts will not cure the patient's problem, but will make the patient less symptomatic for a period of time.

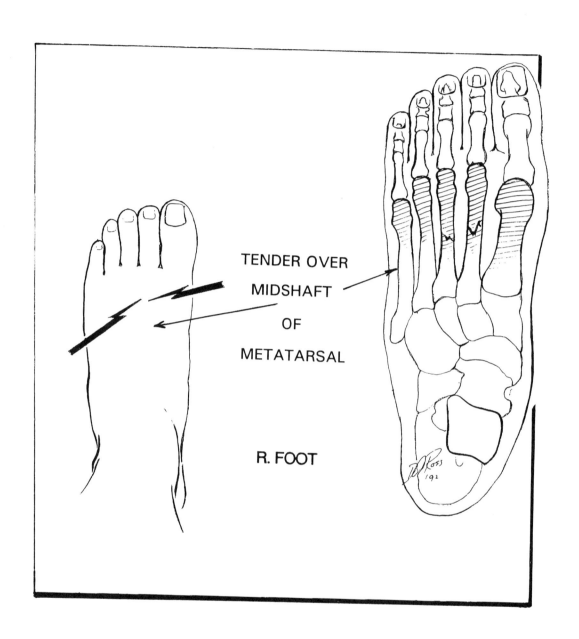

TENDER OVER
MIDSHAFT
OF
METATARSAL

R. FOOT

METATARSAL STRESS FRACTURES

- Stress fractures are usually due to fatigued muscles caused by training errors, not weak bones. On occasion, weak bones may play a role in stress fractures especially in amenorrheic female athletes[34] and in rheumatoid patients.[35-37]

- When the intrinsic muscles of the foot are fatigued, the stress fractures of the metatarsal shaft can occur. Stress fractures can also be caused by bony malalignment.

- Pain is along the metatarsal shaft (not in soft tissues).

- X-rays of the foot may be negative for the first month.

- For the first 4 to 6 weeks, the patient is treated with a postoperative shoe or a cast.

- After 5 weeks, treat with either a medial or lateral longitudinal arch support and metatarsal pad to increase transverse metatarsal arch support. Fractures of the 2nd and 3rd shafts require medial wedging and fractures of the 4th and 5th shafts require lateral wedging.

- Must also decrease activity and wear a stiff shoe.

Fractures of the 2nd or 3rd Shafts

If the hindfoot is in valgus:

- Rx: 5° or 9° medial hindfoot wedge
      Pad proximal to 2nd or 3rd metatarsal head
      Stiff soled shoe
      1 mm heel height

If the hindfoot is in neutral:

- Rx: 0° hindfoot wedge and 5° medial forefoot wedge
      Pad proximal to 2nd or 3rd metatarsal head
      Stiff soled shoe
      1 mm heel height

Fractures of the 4th and 5th Shafts

If the hindfoot is in neutral:

- Rx: 0° hindfoot wedge and 5° lateral forefoot wedge
      Pad proximal to 4th or 5th metatarsal head
      Stiff soled shoe
      1 mm heel height

If the hindfoot is in varus:

- Rx: 5° lateral hindfoot wedge
      Pad proximal to 4th or 5th metatarsal head
      Stiff soled shoe
      1 mm heel height

PART SEVEN

MIDFOOT CONDITIONS

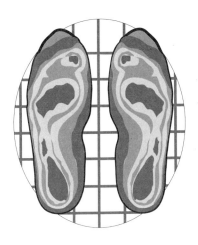

Dorsal Subluxation of the 4th Metatarsocuboid Joint
Abductor Hallucis Myositis
Midfoot Plantar Fasciitis
Accessory Navicular Bone

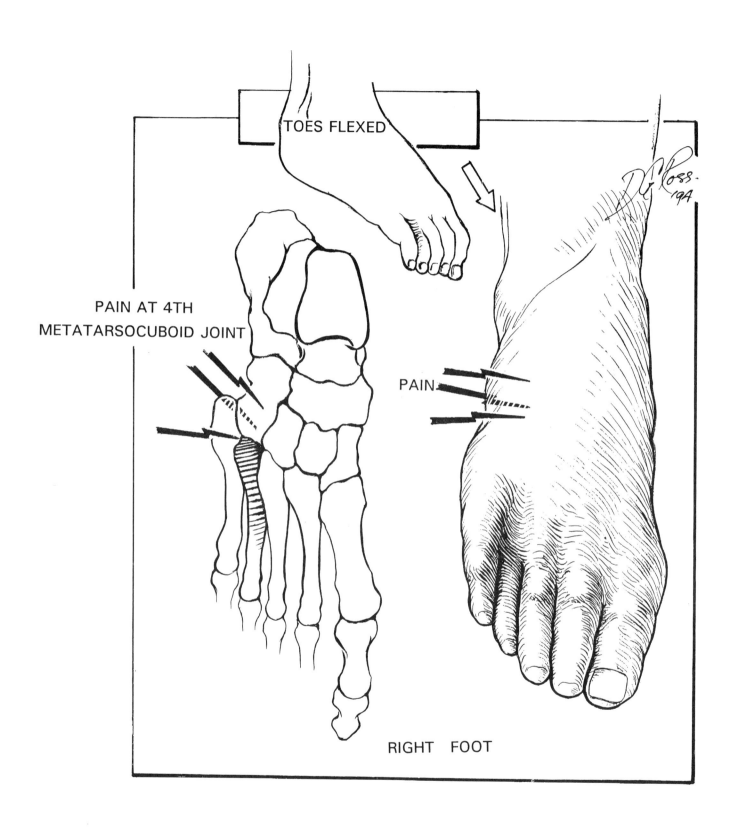

TOES FLEXED

PAIN AT 4TH
METATARSOCUBOID JOINT

PAIN

RIGHT FOOT

56

DORSAL SUBLUXATION OF THE 4TH METATARSOCUBOID JOINT

- This is an uncommon problem. It occurs frequently in ballet dancers but also may occur in heavy patients with tight heel cords.

- These patients complain of foot pain with exertion, walking on hard surfaces, and at the end of the day.

- Physical examination reveals tenderness over the 4th metatarsocuboid joint or the cuboid bone.

- Examination also reveals a lack of prominence of the 4th metatarsal head when the lesser toes are curled (Figure, page 56).[38]

- Most patients are improved with the orthotic prescription written below after reduction of the cuboid by the cuboid squeeze technique. The cuboid squeeze is performed with the foot and ankle in maximum plantar flexion followed by dorsal pressure on the cuboid with the examiner's thumbs.

If the hindfoot is in neutral:

- Rx: 0° hindfoot wedge and 5° lateral forefoot wedge
    Pad proximal to the 4th metatarsal head
    Toe gripping exercises and calf stretching
    1 mm heel height

If the hindfoot is in varus:

- Rx: 5° lateral hindfoot wedge
    Pad proximal to the 4th metatarsal head
    1 mm heel height

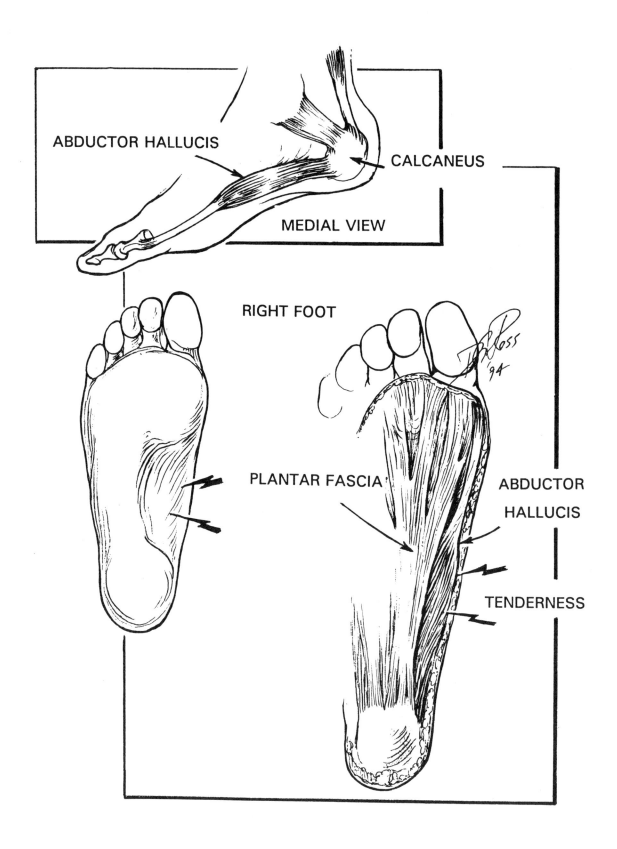

ABDUCTOR HALLUCIS

CALCANEUS

MEDIAL VIEW

RIGHT FOOT

PLANTAR FASCIA

ABDUCTOR HALLUCIS

TENDERNESS

58

ABDUCTOR HALLUCIS MYOSITIS

- This is an overuse syndrome.

- The condition is most common in males in the third decade of life.

- These patients complain of pain in the foot with sprinting.

- Physical examination shows tenderness in the soft tissue of the medial longitudinal arch. The tenderness is not found at the posterior tibial insertion in the navicular, but in the muscle belly of the abductor hallucis.

If the hindfoot is in valgus:

- Rx: 5° or 9° medial hindfoot wedge
    Daily calf stretching
    1 mm heel height

If the hindfoot is in neutral:

- Rx: 0° hindfoot wedge
    5° medial forefoot wedge
    1 mm heel height

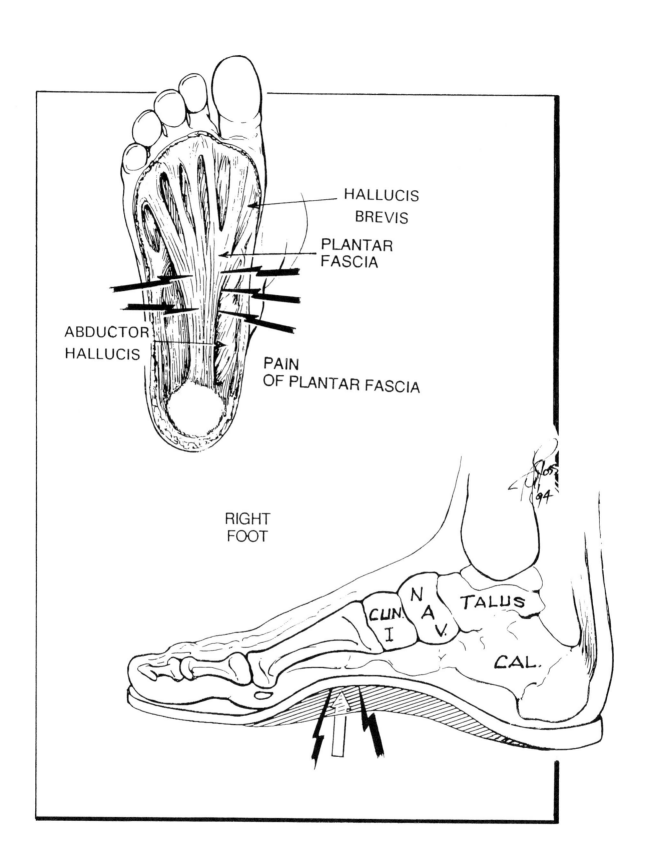

HALLUCIS BREVIS

PLANTAR FASCIA

ABDUCTOR HALLUCIS

PAIN OF PLANTAR FASCIA

RIGHT FOOT

CUN. I

N A V.

TALUS

CAL.

MIDFOOT PLANTAR FASCIITIS

- On occasion, plantar fasciitis occurs in the center of the medial longitudinal arch instead of at the calcaneal insertion of the plantar fascia.

- Pain and tenderness are located in the non–weight-bearing portion of the plantar surface of the foot.

- See the discussion of plantar fasciitis in the hindfoot on page 67.

- Orthotic treatment is keyed to the position of the hindfoot plus the mobility of the 1st ray.

If the hindfoot is in valgus:

- Rx: 5° or 9° medial hindfoot wedge
      1 mm heel height

If the hindfoot is in neutral:

- Rx: 0° hindfoot wedge
      5° medial forefoot wedge
      1 mm heel height

If the hindfoot is in neutral with hypermobile 1st ray:

- Rx: 0° hindfoot wedge
      5° lateral forefoot wedge
      1 mm heel height

If the hindfoot is in varus:

- Rx: 5° lateral hindfoot wedge
      1 mm heel height

All may require 9 mm heel height early in treatment due to tight heel cords.

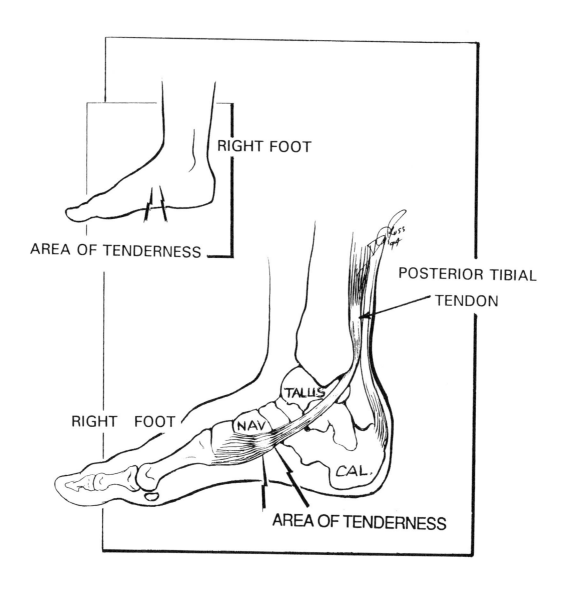

RIGHT FOOT

AREA OF TENDERNESS

POSTERIOR TIBIAL
TENDON

RIGHT FOOT

TALUS

NAV

CAL.

AREA OF TENDERNESS

ACCESSORY NAVICULAR BONE

- An accessory navicular bone is a congenital anomaly of the foot.[39]

- In some patients, the accessory bone causes localized pain because it rubs against the shoe. In these cases, making changes in shoewear to accommodate the osseous bump is all that is necessary.

- In these cases, support for the medial longitudinal arch is required. In acutely painful cases, a cast is required for 6 weeks.

- As with any pathology of the medial longitudinal arch, calf stretching is needed.

- Most patients with this anomaly are asymptomatic. Of the 22 patients I have seen with symptomatic accessory naviculae, only four have required surgery.

If the hindfoot is in valgus:

- Rx: 5° or 9° medial hindfoot wedge after casting or if casting is not required
     Calf stretching is needed to reduce stresses on the medial longitudinal arch
     1 mm heel once calf is stretched out

If the hindfoot is in neutral:

- Rx: 0° hindfoot wedge
     5° medial forefoot wedge
     Calf stretching is needed to reduce stresses on the medial longitudinal arch
     1 mm heel once calf is stretched out

May require 9 mm heel height initially.

PART EIGHT

HINDFOOT AND GLOBAL FOOT CONDITIONS

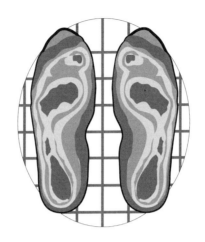

Plantar Fasciitis (heel pain)
Anterior Tibial Tendinitis
Posterior Tibial Tendinitis
Flexor Hallucis Longus Tendinitis
Tarsal Tunnel Syndrome
Achilles Tendinitis
Calcaneal Apophysitis
Global Foot Conditions

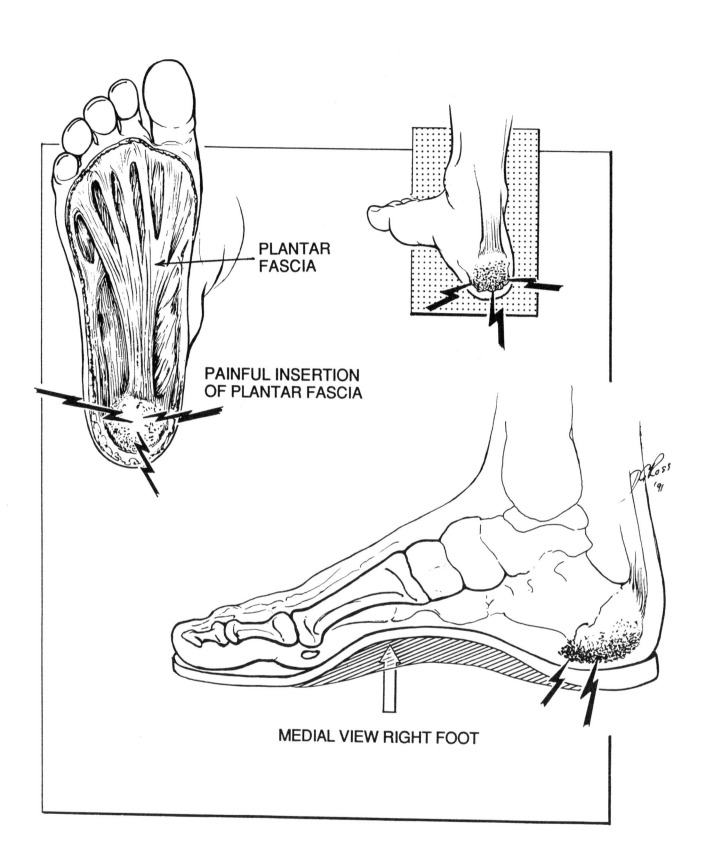

PLANTAR
FASCIA

PAINFUL INSERTION
OF PLANTAR FASCIA

MEDIAL VIEW RIGHT FOOT

PLANTAR FASCIITIS
(HEEL PAIN)

- Inflammation of the origin of the plantar fascia.

- Probably not related to heel spurs. Fifteen percent of normal feet have heel spurs; 50% of painful heels have no spurs.[40]

- The plantar fascia is one of the six major structures supporting the medial longitudinal arch. Therefore, the condition is helped by decreasing hind- and midfoot pronation with a medial wedge.

- Is all the treatment needed? No. Research documents strength and flexibility deficits in the posterior calf and foot in patients who are affected by plantar fasciitis.[41] The calf muscles work against the medial longitudinal arch (Figure, page 10) and need to be stretched at least 1 minute, five times per day.

- Injections are seldom indicated unless only short-term goals are desired by a patient or an athlete.

- Orthotic treatment is keyed to the position of the hindfoot and the mobility of the 1st ray.

If the hindfoot is in valgus:

- Rx: 5° or 9° medial hindfoot wedge
    1 mm heel height

If the hindfoot is in neutral:

- Rx: 0° hindfoot wedge
    5° medial forefoot wedge
    1 mm heel height

If the hindfoot is in neutral with hypermobile 1st ray:

- Rx: 0° hindfoot wedge
    5° lateral forefoot wedge
    1 mm heel height

If the hindfoot is in varus:

- Rx: 5° lateral hindfoot wedge
    1 mm heel height

May require 9 mm heel height early in treatment due to tight heel cords.

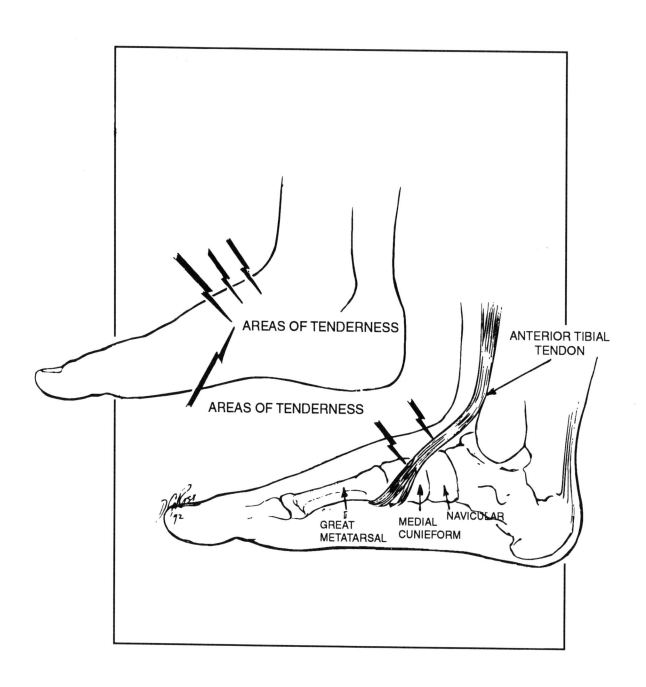

AREAS OF TENDERNESS

AREAS OF TENDERNESS

ANTERIOR TIBIAL
TENDON

GREAT
METATARSAL

MEDIAL
CUNIEFORM

NAVICULAR

ANTERIOR TIBIAL TENDINITIS

- Painful inflammation of the anterior tibial tendon.

- Tenderness is found over the tendon, especially at the insertion.

- The anterior tibial tendon helps hold up the medial longitudinal arch (Figure, page 10).

- Therefore, treatment should support the medial longitudinal arch.

- Treat with medial hindfoot wedge. Patient should also stretch the calf and strengthen the anterior tibial tendon.

- Resistant cases may require temporary immobilization.

If the hindfoot is in valgus:

- Rx: 5° or 9° medial hindfoot wedge
     1 mm heel height

If the hindfoot is in neutral:

- Rx: 0° hindfoot wedge
     5° medial forefoot wedge
     1 mm heel height

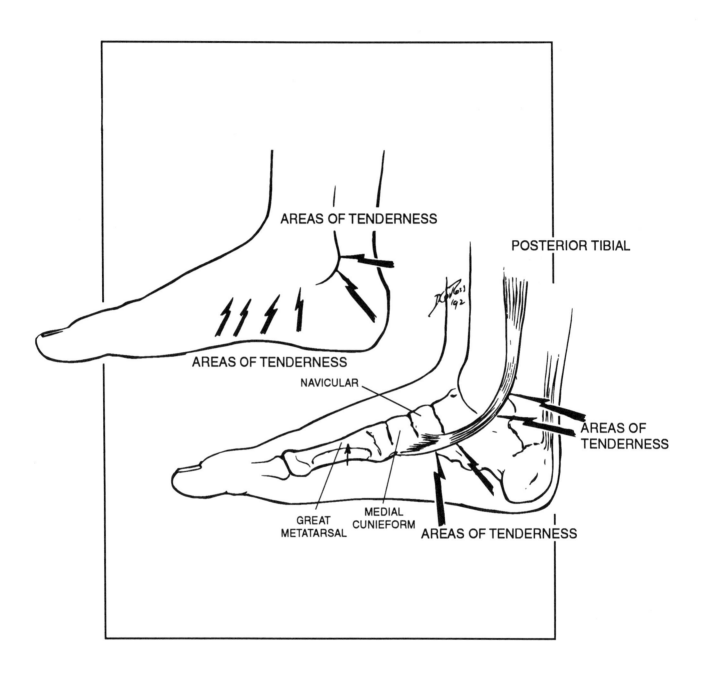

AREAS OF TENDERNESS

POSTERIOR TIBIAL

AREAS OF TENDERNESS

NAVICULAR

AREAS OF TENDERNESS

GREAT METATARSAL

MEDIAL CUNIEFORM

AREAS OF TENDERNESS

POSTERIOR TIBIAL TENDINITIS

- Painful inflammation of the posterior tibial tendon.

- Physical examination usually reveals tenderness at the navicular insertion or just behind the medial malleolus along the tendon.

- In younger patients, this is caused by an overuse of the posterior tibialis or relative weakness of this muscle. In older patients, posterior tibial tendinitis is caused by degeneration of the tendon and is less responsive to conservative treatment.

- Treat with stretching the calf, strengthening the posterior tibialis, and a medial hindfoot wedge.

- Cast immobilization may be required in severe cases.

- Rx: 5° or 9° medial hindfoot wedge
    3 mm heel height (may require 9 mm heel height temporarily)

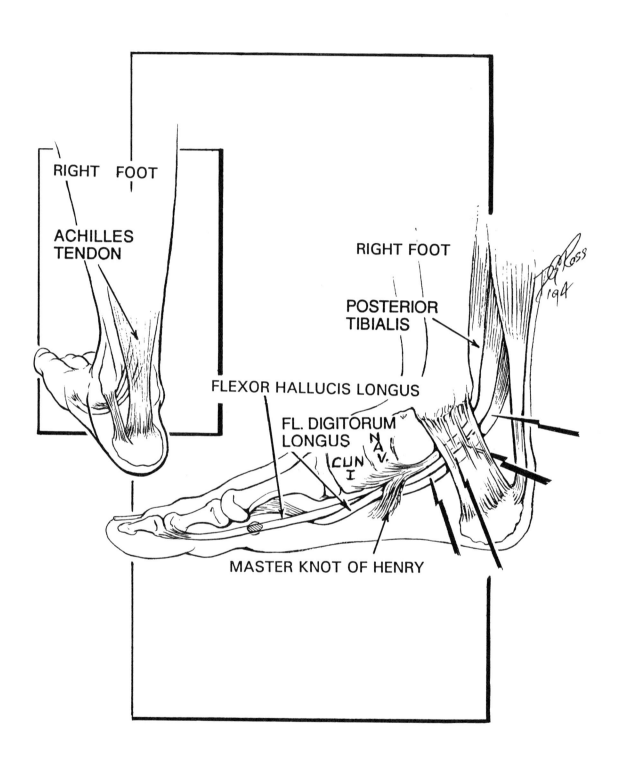

RIGHT FOOT

ACHILLES
TENDON

RIGHT FOOT

POSTERIOR
TIBIALIS

FLEXOR HALLUCIS LONGUS

FL. DIGITORUM
LONGUS

N
A.
V.

CUN
I

MASTER KNOT OF HENRY

FLEXOR HALLUCIS LONGUS TENDINITIS

- Patients with tendinitis of the flexor hallucis longus present with posterior ankle pain extending just distal to the talus.[42] The pain and tenderness do not extend as far as Henry's knot.[43]

- This condition is a common problem in ballet dancers and less so in runners.

- The flexor hallucis longus can rupture.[42]

- Surgery is required if symptoms persist, in which case the tendon sheath requires surgical release. Surgery is also indicated if the tendon ruptures.

- This problem is aggravated by pronation (Figure, page 10).

If the hindfoot is in valgus:

- Rx: 5° or 9° medial hindfoot wedge
      3 mm heel height (may require 9 mm heel height temporarily)
      Calf stretching
      Slow gentle flexor hallucis longus strengthening
      Patients need to change activity

If the hindfoot is in neutral:

- Rx: 0° hindfoot wedge
      5° medial forefoot wedge
      3 mm heel height (may require 9 mm heel height temporarily)

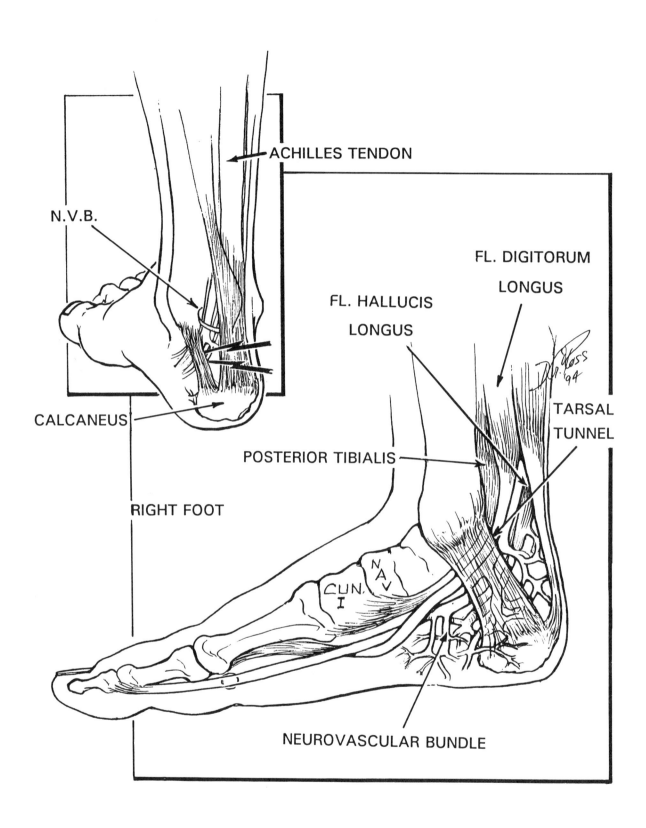

ACHILLES TENDON

N.V.B.

FL. DIGITORUM
LONGUS

FL. HALLUCIS
LONGUS

CALCANEUS

TARSAL
TUNNEL

POSTERIOR TIBIALIS

N
A
V

CUN.
I

RIGHT FOOT

NEUROVASCULAR BUNDLE

TARSAL TUNNEL SYNDROME

- Rare syndrome. Hard to diagnose and treat.

- Diagnose with palpable tenderness and/or tingling over the posterior tibial nerve (between flexor digitorum and flexor hallucis longus tendons).

- Most definitive diagnostic tool is the nerve conduction study across the tarsal tunnel. This test is not infallible and many false negative results are seen (Cimino, personal communication, 1993).

- This is the only medial hindfoot problem that is treated with a lateral hindfoot wedge.

- If hindfoot is already in valgus, diagnosis should be rechecked. This may be an entrapment of the lateral plantar nerve, which does occur with pronation, and is treated with a medial hindfoot wedge.[44]

- The above point regarding the valgus hindfoot vs. the varus hindfoot in tarsal tunnel syndrome is somewhat controversial. Many excellent reviews of tarsal tunnel syndrome suggest that it is due to a valgus deformity of the hindfoot.[45] According to this theory, the posterior tibial nerve is stretched by a valgus hindfoot as it goes around the foot. This makes intuitive sense. Consequently, the first four cases of tarsal tunnel syndrome were treated with medial wedges. All became worse or were no better. Subsequently, after studying Radin's 1983 anatomical review of the tarsal tunnel syndrome, which describes the kinking of the posterior tibial nerve in the varus hindfoot, patients have been treated with lateral wedges.[46]

- Currently, a lateral hindfoot wedge is used for this condition to try to put the hindfoot in valgus. If the hindfoot stays in a varus position despite lateral wedging, then the insert will not help much.

- On occasion, the patient may be helped by an injection into the tarsal tunnel.

If the hindfoot is in varus:

- Rx: 5° or 9° lateral hindfoot wedge
    3 mm heel height

If the hindfoot is in neutral:

- Rx: 0° hindfoot wedge
    5° lateral forefoot wedge
    1 mm heel height

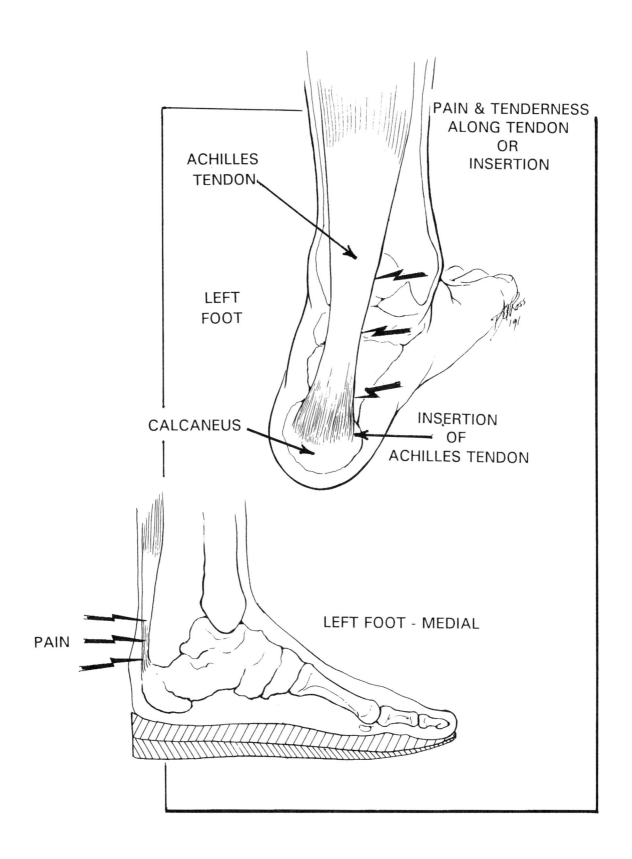

ACHILLES TENDON

PAIN & TENDERNESS ALONG TENDON OR INSERTION

LEFT FOOT

CALCANEUS

INSERTION OF ACHILLES TENDON

PAIN

LEFT FOOT - MEDIAL

ACHILLES TENDINITIS

- Painful inflammation of the Achilles tendon due to:
  Inadequate strength of the gastroc-soleus complex
  Overuse of the gastroc-soleus complex
  Degeneration of the tendon

- Diagnosed by tenderness of the tendon, either at the insertion on the calcaneus or anywhere along its course.

- Heel needs to be elevated to decrease stress.

- Treat with heel height of 9 mm bilaterally and a medial hindfoot wedge.

- Also begin slow strengthening and stretching of the gastroc-soleus complex.

- Patients may require cast immobilization.

If the hindfoot is in valgus:

- Rx: 5° or 9° medial hindfoot wedges
  9 mm heel height

If the hindfoot is in neutral:

- Rx: 0° hindfoot wedge
  5° medial forefoot wedge
  9 mm heel height

If the hindfoot is in varus:

- Rx: 5° lateral forefoot wedge
  9 mm heel height

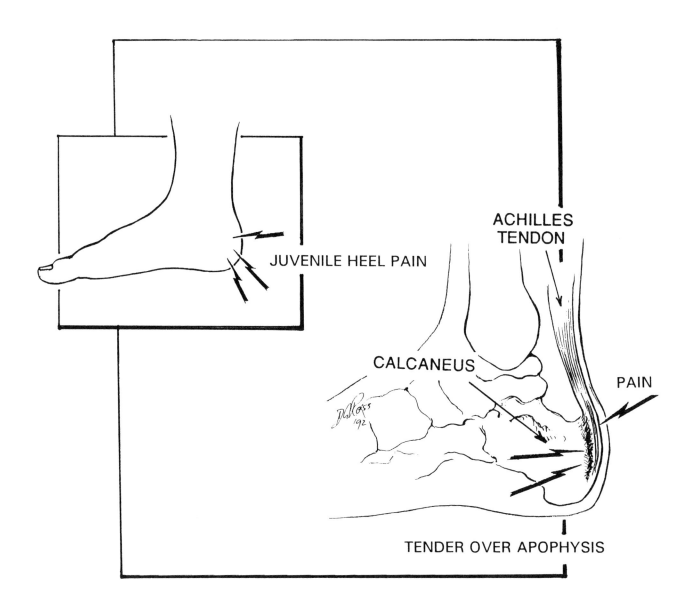

JUVENILE HEEL PAIN

ACHILLES TENDON

CALCANEUS

PAIN

TENDER OVER APOPHYSIS

CALCANEAL APOPHYSITIS

- Occurs in juveniles.

- Pathomechanics for calcaneal apophysitis are exactly the same as for Achilles tendinitis.

- However, in apophysitis, the weak link is the attachment of the calcaneal apophysis to the calcaneus (not in the tendon to the calcaneus, as in Achilles tendinitis).

- Treat with 9 mm heel height.

- May require cast immobilization.

If the hindfoot is in valgus:

- Rx: 5° or 9° medial hindfoot wedge
      9 mm heel height

If the hindfoot is in neutral:

- Rx: 0° hindfoot wedge
      5° medial forefoot wedge
      9 mm heel height

If the hindfoot is in varus:

- Rx: 5° lateral hindfoot wedge
      9 mm heel height

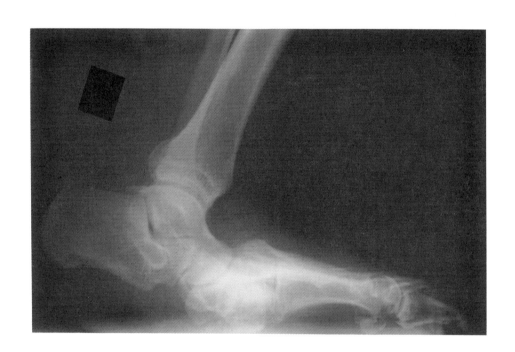

GLOBAL FOOT CONDITIONS

- Several diseases affect the skin, vascular supply, and the entire foot.

- The three most common global foot conditions are: rheumatoid arthritis, diabetes mellitus, and lower extremity arterial insufficiency.

- These patients require thicker, softer inserts.

- Treat with soft insoles 4 mm thick and a medial wedge. Some diabetics may not tolerate the EVA material and require something with more cushion and thickness. (Also, write one of the three diagnoses above on to the prescription.)

- Severe deformity (either from trauma or systemic disease) may require that a foot be digitized in a non–weight-bearing position. All other conditions in this manual are treated with inserts patterned from a weight-bearing foot or a partially weight-bearing foot.

- Rx: Soft orthotic material, 4 mm thick
    5° or 9° medial hindfoot wedge
    1 mm heel height
    Make orthotic in non–weight-bearing position if there is severe bony prominence in the
        medial longitudinal arch
    Extra-depth shoes are also helpful

PART NINE

ANKLE AND SHIN CONDITIONS

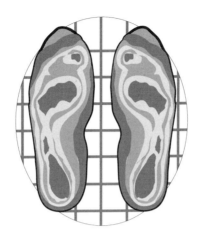

Lateral Soft Tissue Ankle Impingement
(pain between talus and fibula)
Transchondral Fractures/Osteochondritis Dissecans
of the Talus (medial dome)
Shin Splints (anterior tibial myositis)
Flexor Digitorum Longus Myositis

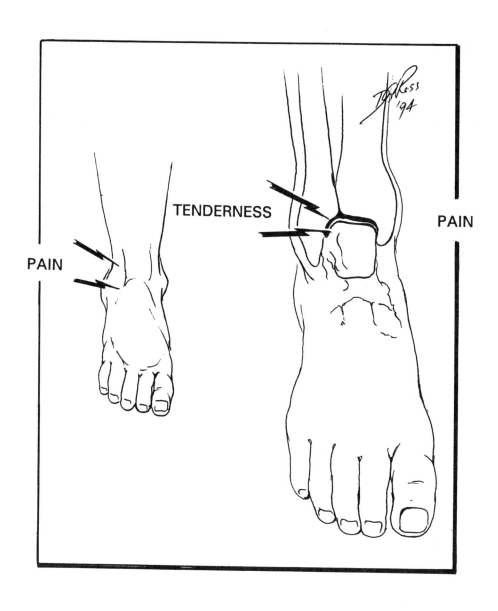

LATERAL SOFT TISSUE ANKLE IMPINGEMENT
(PAIN BETWEEN TALUS AND FIBULA)

- Some patients have chronic pain in the corner of the ankle between the fibula, talus, and tibia following an ankle sprain. They have tenderness of the antero-lateral gutter of the ankle.[47]

- This pain is due to the pinching of strands of ligament and hypertrophic synovium in the above described area.

- If the pain and tenderness is located between the tibia and fibula only, and/or it is reproduced by external rotation of the ankle, then a syndesmotic injury is present rather than an impingement syndrome.[48] Computer-generated inserts will not help patients with even a mild syndesmotic injury.

- Treat ankle impingement with a medial hindfoot wedge before arthroscopy, especially if the patient is pronated.

- Rx: 5° or 9° medial hindfoot wedge
      3 mm to 4 mm heel height*

*Since the anterior talus is wider than the posterior talus, a higher heel decreases the compression between the fibula and talus during weight-bearing.

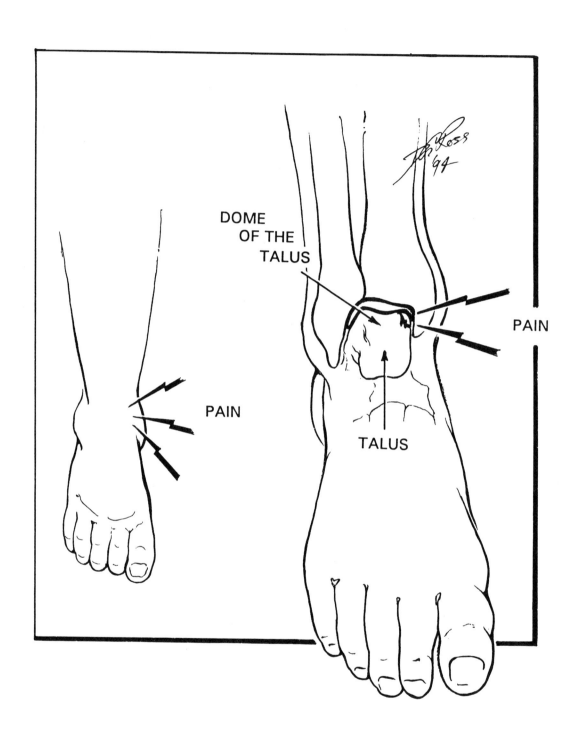

DOME
OF THE
TALUS

TALUS

PAIN

PAIN

TRANSCHONDRAL FRACTURES/
OSTEOCHONDRITIS DISSECANS OF THE TALUS
(MEDIAL DOME)

- Transchondral fractures of the dome of the talus were once believed to be caused by idiopathic avascular necrosis. The opinion now is that the condition is caused by trauma—either single or repeated trauma.[49]

- Lesions on the lateral dome are most likely caused by a single trauma, while medial dome lesions are caused by repetitive or unrecognized trauma.[50]

- Patients with transchondral fractures of the medial dome present with medial ankle pain and no history of a single trauma. Tenderness is palpable anterior or inferior to the medial malleolus. Diagnosis is made with x-rays, MRI, or CT scan.

- Initial treatment is non–weight-bearing cast immobilization for 6 weeks.

- If this treatment fails, then arthroscopy is indicated, followed by 2 months on crutches.

- Even 2 months after arthroscopy, about half these patients still have some medial ankle swelling and tenderness. In these patients, a medial hindfoot wedge is symptomatically helpful. The reason for this symptom reduction is that the compression in this lesion occurs between the talus and the medial malleolus, not the talus and the tibial pilon.*

- In addition, alterations in heel height affect the portion of the talus articulating with the tibia during single stance weight-bearing.

- Rx: 5° or 9° medial hindfoot wedge
    1 mm heel height with posterior dome lesion
    3 mm or 9 mm heel height with anterior dome lesion

*Patients treated with lateral hindfoot wedges became much more symptomatic.

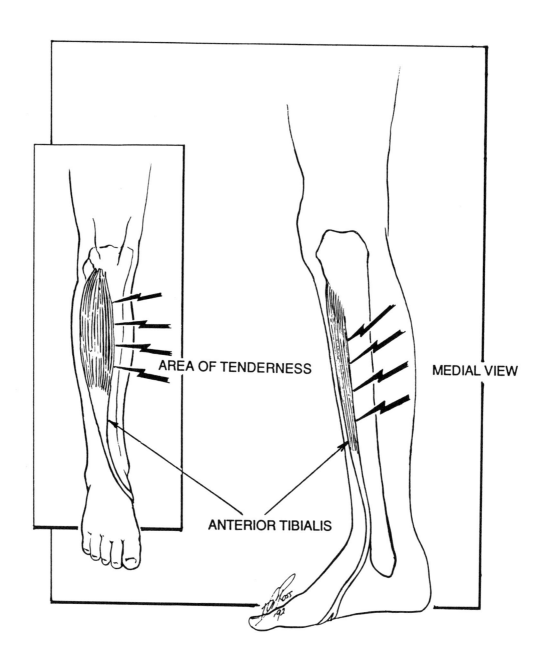

AREA OF TENDERNESS

MEDIAL VIEW

ANTERIOR TIBIALIS

SHIN SPLINTS
(ANTERIOR TIBIAL MYOSITIS)

- Shin splints are a painful inflammation of the origin of the anterior tibialis muscle.

- It is caused by relative weakness or overuse of the anterior tibialis and tightness of the calf muscles.

- Since the anterior tibialis helps support the medial longitudinal arch, and since tibial stress syndromes are significantly reduced by wearing insoles, insoles that support the arch will help this condition.[51]

- Treat with a medial longitudinal arch support

- Encourage anterior tibialis strengthening and gastrocnemius soleus stretching.

If the hindfoot is in valgus:

- Rx: 5° or 9° medial hindfoot wedge
    1 mm heel height

If the hindfoot is in neutral:

- Rx: 0° hindfoot wedge
    5° medial forefoot wedge
    1 mm heel height

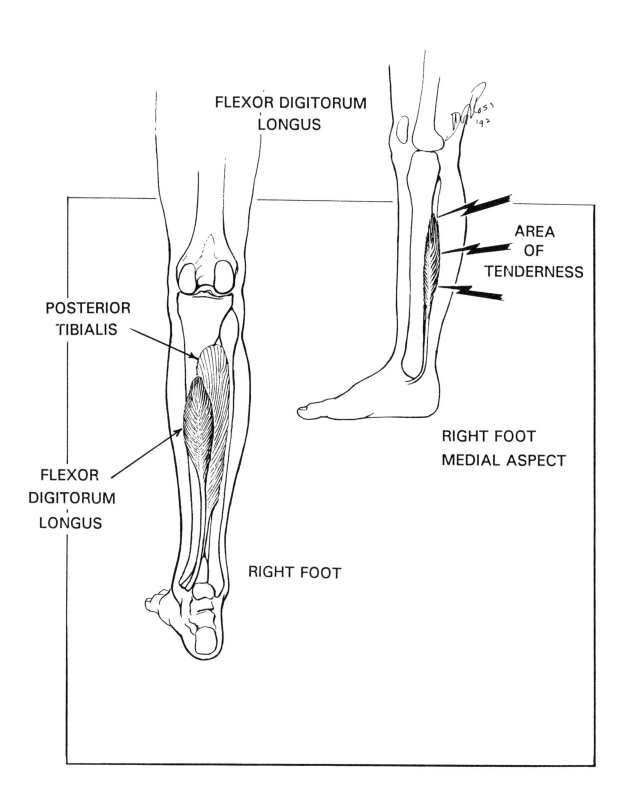

FLEXOR DIGITORUM
LONGUS

POSTERIOR
TIBIALIS

FLEXOR
DIGITORUM
LONGUS

RIGHT FOOT

AREA
OF
TENDERNESS

RIGHT FOOT
MEDIAL ASPECT

90

FLEXOR DIGITORUM LONGUS MYOSITIS

- Flexor digitorum longus myositis is a painful overuse syndrome of the origin of the flexor digitorum longus muscle.

- Tenderness is found over the medial distal half of the tibia.

- Frequently, it is a good idea to x-ray the leg to rule out a tibial stress fracture.

- Since the flexor digitorum longus supports the medial longitudinal arch, this condition is treated with medial arch support.

If the hindfoot is in valgus:

- Rx: 5° or 9° medial hindfoot wedge
     3 mm heel height (may require 9 mm heel height temporarily)

If the hindfoot is in neutral:

- Rx: 0° hindfoot wedge
     5° medial forefoot wedge
     3 mm heel height (may require 9 mm heel height temporarily)

PART TEN

KNEE CONDITIONS

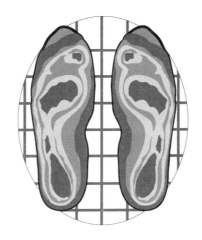

Pes Anserine Bursitis
Chondromalacia Patella (retropatellar pain syndrome)
Iliotibial Band Syndrome
Unicompartmental Knee Arthritis
Popliteal Tendinitis

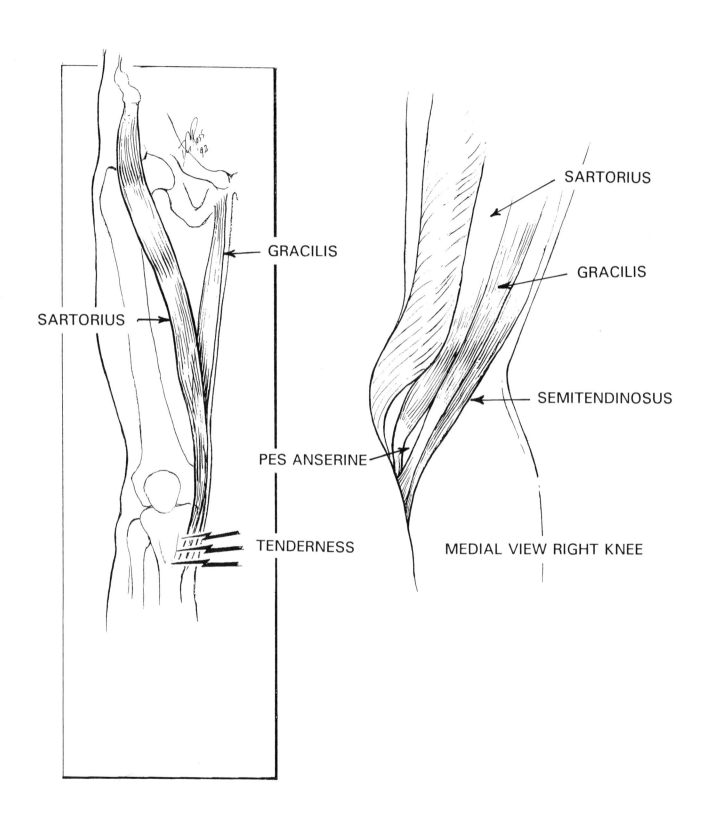

SARTORIUS

GRACILIS

PES ANSERINE

TENDERNESS

SARTORIUS

GRACILIS

SEMITENDINOSUS

MEDIAL VIEW RIGHT KNEE

PES ANSERINE BURSITIS

- This is a painful condition of the medial side of the proximal tibia.

- The inflamed bursa is beneath the three tendons that comprise the pes anserine (sartorius, semitendinosus, and gracilis).

- Decreasing foot pronation with a medial hindfoot wedge will decrease the stretch on these tendons.

- Hamstring stretching, quad strengthening, and avoidance of hills also helps.

- Rx: 5° or 9° medial hindfoot wedge
    1 mm heel height

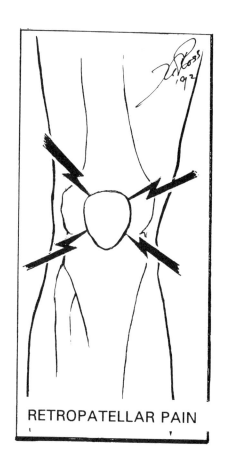

RETROPATELLAR PAIN

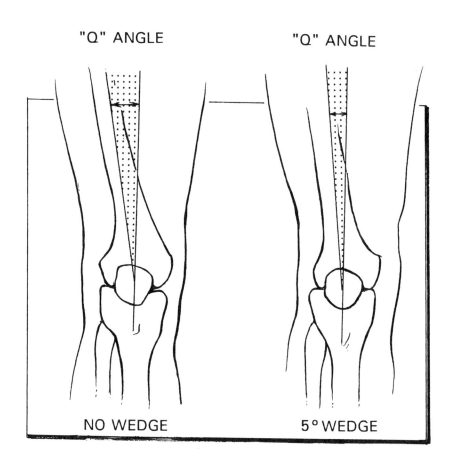

"Q" ANGLE   "Q" ANGLE

NO WEDGE   5° WEDGE

CHONDROMALACIA PATELLA
(RETROPATELLAR PAIN SYNDROME)

- The most common cause of knee pain is chondromalacia patella.

- It is diagnosed by palpating tenderness under either the medial or lateral patellar facet. The rest of the knee exam is basically normal, although there may be a slight effusion.

- Many times the chondromalacia is accompanied with a pronated foot.[17,52] If this is the case, the patient can be helped with a medial hindfoot wedge. The reason for this is that for every degree the foot is supinated, the "Q" angle decreases .44°.[18]

- It has also been shown that soft foot orthotics are effective in decreasing the pain in this syndrome.[53]

If the hindfoot is in valgus:

- Rx: 5° or 9° medial hindfoot wedge
    1 mm heel height

If the hindfoot is in neutral:

- Rx: 0° hindfoot wedge
    5° medial forefoot wedge
    1 mm heel height

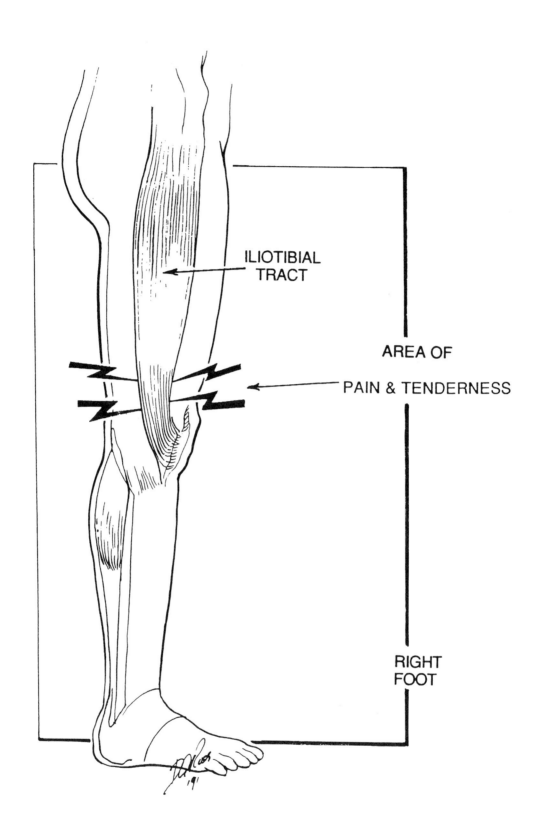

ILIOTIBIAL
TRACT

AREA OF

PAIN & TENDERNESS

RIGHT
FOOT

98

ILIOTIBIAL BAND SYNDROME

- The iliotibial band extends from the pelvis across the lateral aspect of the knee.

- When this region becomes inflamed, the tenderness is usually palpable on the lateral aspect of the knee.

- If the patient has a pronated (flat) foot, the tibia internally rotates and increases the distance the band must travel to its insertion on the proximal tibia. This type of patient is treated with a medial hindfoot wedge.

- If the patient has a cavus foot or a varus heel, the iliotibial band is placed on a stretch. The stretch is decreased with a lateral hindfoot wedge.

If the hindfoot is in valgus:

- Rx: 5° or 9° medial hindfoot wedge
  1 mm heel height

If the hindfoot is in varus:

- Rx: 5° or 9° lateral hindfoot wedge
  1 mm heel height

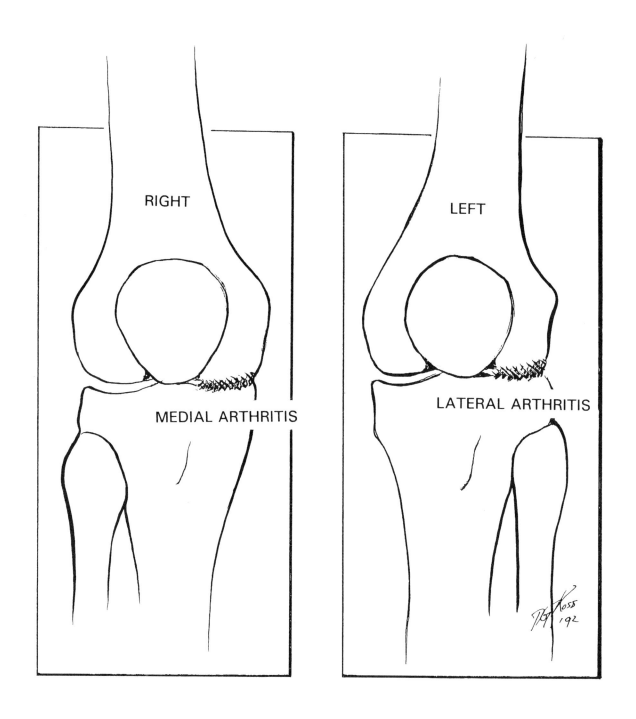

RIGHT

MEDIAL ARTHRITIS

LEFT

LATERAL ARTHRITIS

UNICOMPARTMENTAL KNEE ARTHRITIS

- An orthotic or shoe insert for a patient with unicompartmental knee arthritis can be helpful but really only as an adjunct or temporizing measure.

- Arthritic knee pain is relieved by various anti-inflammatories, walking aids, and eventually surgery. If a patient is not a candidate for any of the above and does not wish to have surgery, then an insert may help.

- For medial compartment arthritis, prescribe a lateral hindfoot wedge. For lateral compartment arthritis, prescribe a medial hindfoot wedge. These wedges will increase some of the weight-bearing forces across the healthy part of the joint.[54-57]

Medial Compartment Knee Arthritis

- Rx: 5° or 9° lateral hindfoot wedge
      1 mm heel height

Lateral Compartment Knee Arthritis

- Rx: 5° or 9° medial hindfoot wedge
      1 mm heel height

If the patient has a severely pronated foot, then the orthotic prescription should be written to treat the foot, not the knee.

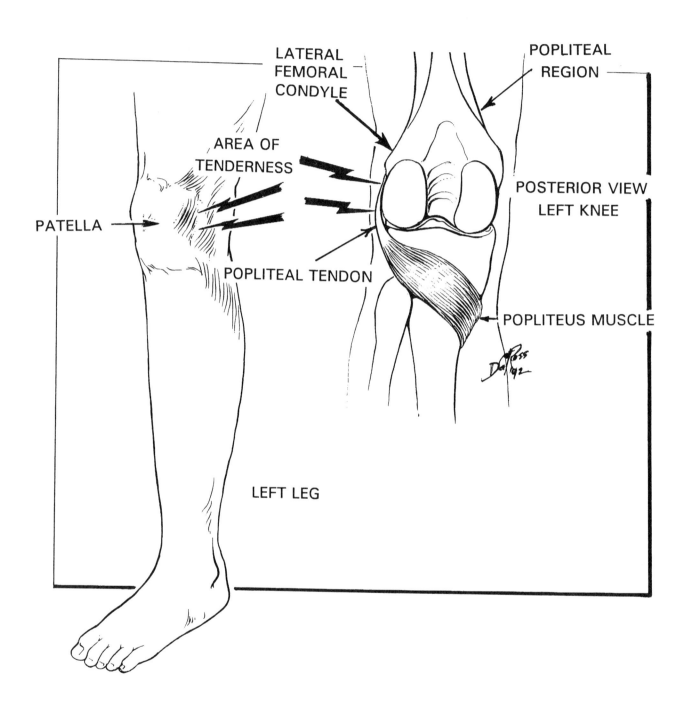

LATERAL
FEMORAL
CONDYLE

POPLITEAL
REGION

AREA OF
TENDERNESS

PATELLA

POSTERIOR VIEW
LEFT KNEE

POPLITEAL TENDON

POPLITEUS MUSCLE

LEFT LEG

POPLITEAL TENDINITIS

- The job of the popliteus muscle is to internally rotate the tibia 10° to 14° (Mann, personal communication, 1992). In addition, the popliteus is the most important posterolateral stabilizer of the knee.[58] This muscle is located behind the knee as shown.

- Popliteal tendinitis is diagnosed by palpating tenderness at the insertion of the popliteus tendon on the lateral femoral condyle near the femoral insertion of the lateral collateral ligament.

- A lateral hindfoot wedge tends to help hold the tibia in an internally rotated position and thereby decrease the stress on the popliteus. A lateral wedge also decreases the varus stresses on the knee which decreases tension on the posterolateral corner of the knee.

- Treat with a 5° lateral hindfoot wed for mild hindfoot varus and a 9° lateral hindfoot wedge if the patient's heel, when viewed from behind, never reaches a valgus or neutral position with the foot fully loaded.

- Rx: 5° or 9° lateral hindfoot wedge
  1 mm heel height

PART ELEVEN

HIP AND LEG LENGTH PROBLEMS

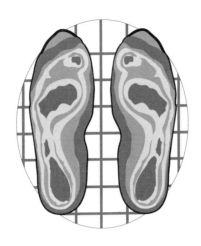

Leg Length Inequality
Trochanteric Bursitis
Gluteus Medius Syndrome

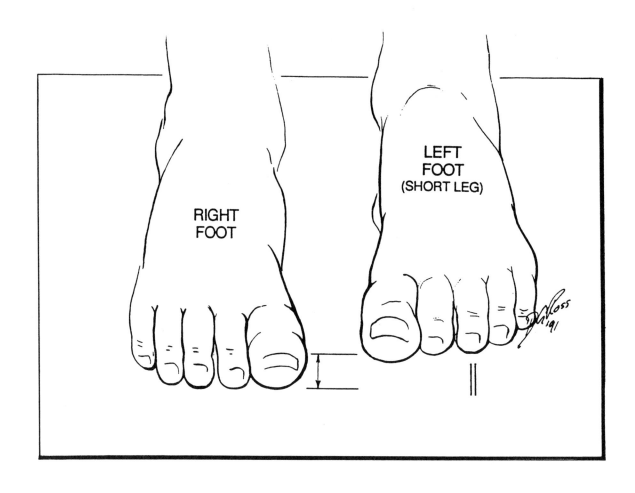

RIGHT FOOT

LEFT FOOT (SHORT LEG)

LEG LENGTH INEQUALITY

- Leg length inequality has been implicated in several painful disorders, including stress fractures, medial knee strain, hyperpronation with resultant plantar fasciitis or patellar subluxation, iliotibial band tendinitis, and lateral knee impingement.[59]

- A leg length discrepancy of as little as 1/4 inch may produce low back pain and lateral hip pain.[12,13] The data are imprecise, however, as to what amount of leg length inequality is clinically significant. Most orthopedic surgeons at this time do not prescribe a lift unless the inequality is 3/4 inch to 1 inch (Ferkel, personal communication, 1993).

- The long leg side can develop low back pain, trochanteric bursitis, or iliotibial tract tendinitis.[1]

- The short leg can develop iliotibial tract tendinitis and lateral ankle impingement.[1]

- The computer-generated orthotic system can add only 3 mm to 9 mm inside the shoe. If more correction is needed, it must be done on the outside of the shoe.

- It is also helpful to add a medial hindfoot wedge to the inserts of both legs.

- Rx: 5° or 9° medial hindfoot wedges bilaterally
  Add 3 mm to 9 mm to heel insert of shorter leg

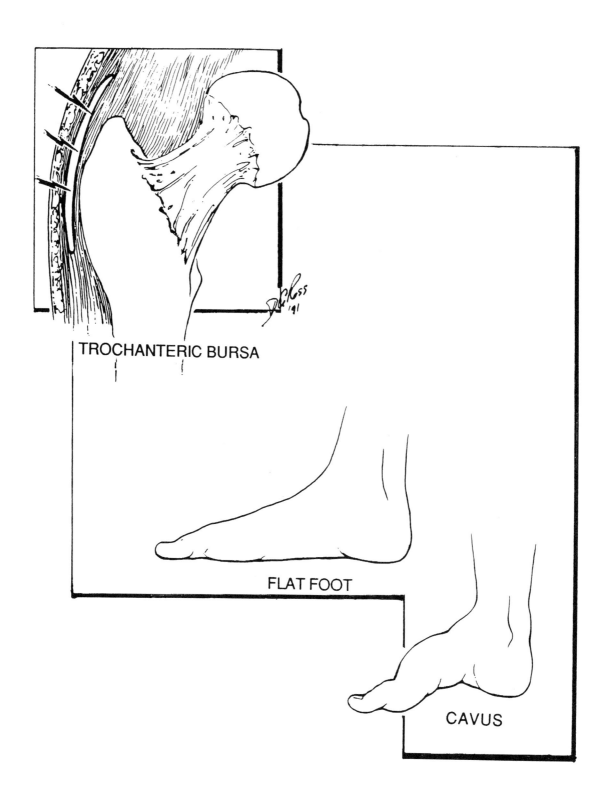

TROCHANTERIC BURSA

FLAT FOOT

CAVUS

108

TROCHANTERIC BURSITIS

- Occurs with pronated feet and in the longer of two legs.[1]

- The pain and tenderness is located over the greater trochanter.

- Check leg lengths.

- Treat any leg length inequality.

- Treat any foot pronation with a medial hindfoot wedge.

- If a cavovarus foot is present, use a lateral hindfoot wedge.

- Patient needs to begin stretching of the iliotibial band.[60]

If the hindfoot is in valgus:

- Rx: 5° or 9° medial hindfoot wedge

If the hindfoot is in varus:

- Rx: 5° or 9° lateral hindfoot wedge

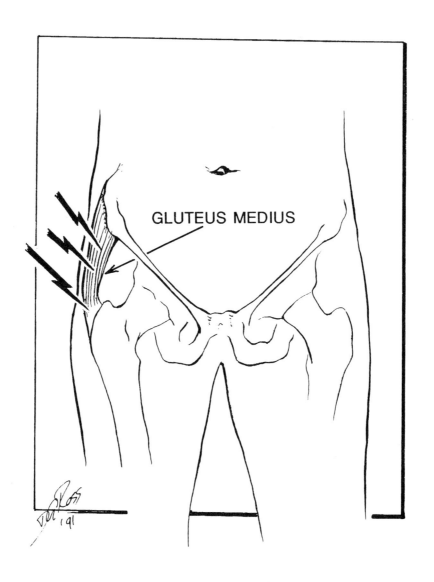

GLUTEUS MEDIUS

GLUTEUS MEDIUS SYNDROME

- Occurs frequently in association with pronated feet.[12,13]

- Pain and tenderness is located above the greater trochanter.

- Treat with a medial hindfoot wedge.

- Check leg lengths.

- These patients also require daily stretching and strengthening of the hip abductors.

- Rx: 5° or 9° medial hindfoot wedge

PART TWELVE

DIAGNOSIS/PRESCRIPTION SUMMARY

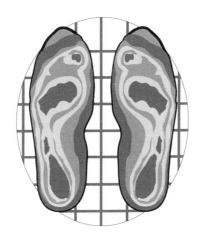

Forefoot Conditions Summary
Midfoot Conditions Summary
Hindfoot and Global Foot Conditions Summary
Ankle and Shin Conditions Summary
Knee Conditions Summary
Hip and Leg Length Problems Summary

FOREFOOT CONDITIONS SUMMARY

All forefoot conditions require 1 mm heel height.

Hammer Toes

Hammer Toes of the 2nd and 3rd Rays

If valgus hindfoot:

- Rx: 5° or 9° medial hindfoot wedge
  Pad proximal to involved toe

If neutral hindfoot:

- Rx: 0° hindfoot wedge plus 5° medial forefoot wedge
  Pad proximal to involved toe

Hammer Toes of the 4th and 5th Rays

If neutral hindfoot:

- Rx: 0° hindfoot wedge plus 5° lateral forefoot wedge
  Pad proximal to involved toe

If varus hindfoot:

- Rx: 5° lateral hindfoot wedge
  Pad proximal to involved toe

Morton's Neuroma

Neuroma Medial to 4th Metatarsal

If valgus hindfoot:

- Rx: 5° or 9° medial hindfoot wedge
  Pad proximal to 2nd or 3rd metatarsal head

If neutral hindfoot:

- Rx: 0° medial forefoot wedge and 5° medial forefoot wedge
  Pad proximal to 2nd or 3rd metatarsal head

Neuroma between the 4th and 5th Metatarsal Heads

If neutral hindfoot:

- Rx: 0° medial hindfoot wedge and 5° lateral forefoot wedge
  Pad proximal to 4th metatarsal head

If varus hindfoot:

- Rx: 5° lateral hindfoot wedge
  Pad proximal to 4th metatarsal head

Metatarsalgia (1st, 2nd, and 3rd metatarsal heads)

If valgus hindfoot:

- Rx: 5° or 9° medial hindfoot wedge
  Pad proximal to the 2nd or 3rd metatarsal head

If neutral hindfoot:

- Rx: 0° hindfoot wedge
    5° medial forefoot wedge
    Pad proximal to 2nd or 3rd metatarsal head

Metatarsalgia (4th and 5th metatarsal heads)

If neutral hindfoot:

- Rx: 0° hindfoot wedge
    5° lateral forefoot wedge
    Pad just proximal to the 4th and 5th heads

If varus hindfoot:

- Rx: 5° hindfoot wedge
    Pad just proximal to the 4th and 5th heads

Sesamoiditis

If valgus hindfoot:

- Rx: 5° or 9° medial hindfoot wedge and pad just proximal to the sesamoids
    Grind out area under sesamoids

If neutral hindfoot:

- Rx: 0° hindfoot wedge
    5° medial forefoot wedge and pad proximal to the sesamoids
    Grind out area under sesamoids

Turf Toe (hyperextension type)

If valgus hindfoot:

- Rx: 5° or 9° medial hindfoot wedge
    Pad proximal to great metatarsal phalangeal joint
    Stiff soled shoe (rocker soled shoe may also help)

If neutral hindfoot:

- Rx: 0° hindfoot wedge
    5° lateral forefoot wedge
    Pad proximal to great metatarsal phalangeal joint
    Stiff soled shoe

Hallux Rigidus

If valgus hindfoot:

- Rx: 5° or 9° medial hindfoot wedge and pad just proximal to the great metatarsal phalangeal
    joint
    Stiff soled shoe

116

If neutral hindfoot:

- Rx: 0° hindfoot wedge
    5° medial forefoot wedge and pad proximal to the great metatarsal phalangeal joint
    Stiff soled shoe

Hallux Valgus

If valgus hindfoot:

- Rx: 5° or 9° medial hindfoot wedge
    Add metatarsal pads if metatarsalgia is present
    Shoe with wide toe box

If neutral hindfoot:

- Rx: 0° hindfoot wedge
    5° medial forefoot wedge
    Metatarsal pad as needed
    Shoes with wide toe box

Metatarsal Stress Fractures

Fractures of the 2nd or 3rd Shafts

If valgus hindfoot:

- Rx: 5° or 9° medial hindfoot wedge
    Pad proximal to 2nd or 3rd metatarsal head
    Stiff soled shoe

If neutral hindfoot:

- Rx: 0° hindfoot wedge and 5° medial forefoot wedge
    Pad proximal to 2nd or 3rd metatarsal head
    Stiff soled shoe

Fractures of the 4th and 5th Shafts

If neutral hindfoot:

- Rx: 0° hindfoot wedge and 5° lateral forefoot wedge
    Pad proximal to 4th or 5th metatarsal head
    Stiff soled shoe

If varus hindfoot:

- Rx: 5° lateral hindfoot wedge
    Pad proximal to 4th or 5th metatarsal head
    Stiff soled shoe

MIDFOOT CONDITIONS SUMMARY

All midfoot conditions require 1 mm heel height.

Dorsal Subluxation of the 4th Metatarsocuboid Joint

If neutral hindfoot:

- Rx: 0° hindfoot wedge and 5° lateral forefoot wedge
    Pad proximal to the 4th metatarsal head
    Toe gripping exercises and calf stretching

If varus hindfoot:

- Rx: 5° lateral hindfoot wedge
    Pad proximal to the 4th metatarsal head

Abductor Hallucis Myositis

If valgus hindfoot:

- Rx: 5° or 9° medial hindfoot wedge
    Daily calf stretching

If neutral hindfoot:

- Rx: 0° hindfoot wedge
    5° medial forefoot wedge

Midfoot Plantar Fasciitis

If valgus hindfoot:

- Rx: 5° or 9° medial hindfoot wedge

If neutral hindfoot:

- Rx: 0° hindfoot wedge
    5° medial forefoot wedge

If neutral hindfoot with hypermobile 1st ray:

- Rx: 0° hindfoot wedge
    5° lateral forefoot wedge

If varus hindfoot:

- Rx: 5° lateral hindfoot wedge

All may require 9 mm heel height early in treatment due to tight heel cords.

Accessory Navicular Bone

If valgus hindfoot:

- Rx: 5° or 9° medial hindfoot wedge after casting or if casting is not required
    Calf stretching is needed to reduce stresses on the medial longitudinal arch
    1 mm heel once calf is stretched out

If neutral hindfoot:

- Rx: 0° hindfoot wedge
    5° medial forefoot wedge
    Calf stretching is needed to reduce stresses on the medial longitudinal arch
    1 mm heel once calf is stretched out

May require 9 mm heel height initially.

HINDFOOT AND GLOBAL FOOT CONDITIONS SUMMARY

Plantar Fasciitis (heel pain)

If valgus hindfoot:

- Rx: 5° or 9° medial hindfoot wedge
    1 mm heel height

If neutral hindfoot:

- Rx: 0° hindfoot wedge
    5° medial forefoot wedge
    1 mm heel height

If neutral hindfoot with hypermobile 1st ray:

- Rx: 0° hindfoot wedge
    5° lateral forefoot wedge
    1 mm heel height

If varus hindfoot:

- Rx: 5° lateral hindfoot wedge
    1 mm heel height

May require 9 mm heel height early in treatment due to tight heel cords.

Anterior Tibial Tendinitis

If valgus hindfoot:

- Rx: 5° or 9° medial hindfoot wedge
    1 mm heel height

If neutral hindfoot:

- Rx: 0° hindfoot wedge
    5° medial forefoot wedge
    1 mm heel height

Posterior Tibial Tendinitis

- Rx: 5° or 9° medial hindfoot wedge
    3 mm heel height (may require 9 mm heel height temporarily)

Flexor Hallucis Longus Tendinitis

If valgus hindfoot:

- Rx: 5° or 9° medial hindfoot wedge
    3 mm heel height (may require 9 mm heel height temporarily)
    Calf stretching
    Slow gentle flexor hallucis longus strengthening
    Patients need to change activity

If neutral hindfoot:

- Rx: 0° hindfoot wedge
    5° medial forefoot wedge
    3 mm heel height (may require 9 mm heel height temporarily)

Tarsal Tunnel Syndrome

If varus hindfoot:

- Rx: 5° or 9° lateral hindfoot wedge
    3 mm heel height

If neutral hindfoot:

- Rx: 0° hindfoot wedge
    5° lateral forefoot wedge
    1 mm heel height

Achilles Tendinitis

If valgus hindfoot:

- Rx: 5° or 9° medial hindfoot wedges
    9 mm heel height

If neutral hindfoot:

- Rx: 0° hindfoot wedge
    5° medial forefoot wedge
    9 mm heel height

If varus hindfoot:

- Rx: 5° lateral forefoot wedge
    9 mm heel height

Calcaneal Apophysitis

If valgus hindfoot:

- Rx: 5° or 9° medial hindfoot wedge
    9 mm heel height

If neutral hindfoot:

- Rx: 0° hindfoot wedge
    5° medial forefoot wedge
    9 mm heel height

If varus hindfoot:

- Rx: 5° lateral hindfoot wedge
    9 mm heel height

Global Foot Conditions

Rheumatoid, Diabetic, Dysvascular

- Rx: Soft orthotic material, 4 mm thick
    5° or 9° medial hindfoot wedge
    1 mm heel height
    Make orthotic in non–weight-bearing position if there is severe bony prominence in the
        medial longitudinal arch
    Extra-depth shoes are also helpful

ANKLE AND SHIN CONDITIONS SUMMARY

Lateral Soft Tissue Ankle Impingement (pain between talus and fibula)

- Rx: 5° or 9° medial hindfoot wedge
    3 mm to 4 mm heel height

Transchondral Fractures/Osteochondritis Dissecans of the Talus (medial dome)

- Rx: 5° or 9° medial hindfoot wedge
    1 mm heel height with posterior dome lesion
    3 mm or 9 mm heel height with anterior dome lesion

Shin Splints (anterior tibial myositis)

If valgus hindfoot:

- Rx: 5° or 9° medial hindfoot wedge
    1 mm heel height

If neutral hindfoot:

- Rx: 0° hindfoot wedge
    5° medial forefoot wedge
    1 mm heel height

Flexor Digitorum Longus Myositis

If valgus hindfoot:

- Rx: 5° or 9° medial hindfoot wedge
    3 mm heel height (may require 9 mm heel height temporarily)

If neutral hindfoot:

- Rx: 0° hindfoot wedge
    5° medial forefoot wedge
    3 mm heel height (may require 9 mm heel height temporarily)

KNEE CONDITIONS SUMMARY

All knee conditions require 1 mm heels.

Pes Anserine Bursitis

- Rx: 5° or 9° medial hindfoot wedge

Chondromalacia Patella (retropatellar pain syndrome)

If valgus hindfoot:

- Rx: 5° or 9° medial hindfoot wedge

If neutral hindfoot:

- Rx: 0° hindfoot wedge
    5° medial forefoot wedge

Iliotibial Band Syndrome

If valgus hindfoot:

- Rx: 5° or 9° medial hindfoot wedge

If varus hindfoot:

- Rx: 5° or 9° lateral hindfoot wedge

Unicompartmental Knee Arthritis

Medial Compartment Knee Arthritis

- Rx: 5° or 9° lateral hindfoot wedge

Lateral Compartment Knee Arthritis

- Rx: 5° or 9° medial hindfoot wedge

If the patient has a severely pronated foot, then the orthotic prescription should be written to treat the foot, not the knee.

Popliteal Tendinitis

- Rx: 5° or 9° lateral hindfoot wedge

HIP AND LEG LENGTH PROBLEMS SUMMARY

Leg Length Inequality

- Rx: 5° or 9° medial hindfoot wedges bilaterally

    Add 3 mm to 9 mm to heel insert of shorter leg

Trochanteric Bursitis

If valgus hindfoot:

- Rx: 5° or 9° medial hindfoot wedge

If varus hindfoot:

- Rx: 5° or 9° lateral hindfoot wedge

Gluteus Medius Syndrome

- Rx: 5° or 9° medial hindfoot wedge

REFERENCES

1. Baxter DE. The foot in running. In: Mann RA, ed. *Surgery of the Foot.* St. Louis, MO: CV Mosby; 1986:509.
2. Stipe P. The effects of orthotics on rearfoot movement in running. *Nike Newsletter.* 1983;2:3.
3. Dressendorfer RH, Wade CD, Frederick EC. Effect of shoe cushioning on the development of reticulocytosis in distance runners. *Amer J Sports Medicine.* 1992;20(2):212-216.
4. Falsetti ML, Burke ER, Feld R, Fredericks EC, Ratering C. Hematological variations after endurance running and hard- and soft-soled running shoes. *Physicians and Sportsmedicine.* 1983;11:118-127.
5. Mann RA. *Surgery of the Foot.* 5th ed. St. Louis, MO: CV Mosby; 1986:16.
6. Clark TE, Frederick EC, Hamill CL. The effect of shoe design upon rearfoot movement in running. *Med Sci Sports Exerc.* 1983;15(5):376-381.
7. Sanderson DJ, Taunton JE. *Evaluation of thermoplastic and EVA orthotics in the control of rearfoot motion during running.* University of British Columbia. In press.
8. McMahan JO. Proper footwear for play and the fitting of painful deformed feet. *American Academy of Orthopedic Surgeons Symposium on the Foot and Ankle.* St. Louis, MO: CV Mosby; 1983:50.
9. Lutter LD. *Athletes' Heel Pain.* Presented at the meeting of the American Orthopedic Foot Society. Anaheim, Calif; March 1983.
10. Bordelon RL. *Surgical and Conservative Foot Care.* Thorofare, NJ: SLACK Inc; 1988:177.
11. Brody DM. Techniques in the evaluation and treatment of the injured runner. *Orthop Clin North Am.* 1982;13:3.
12. Brody D. Rehabilitation of the injured runner. *American Academy of Orthopedic Surgeons' Instructional Course Lecture.* St. Louis, MO: CV Mosby; 1984:270.
13. Schuster. Secondary citation in Brody D. Rehabilitation of the injured runner. *American Academy of Orthopedic Surgeons' Instructional Course Lecture.* St. Louis, MO: CV Mosby; 1958.
14. Hamilton JJ, Ziemer LK. Functional anatomy of the human ankle and foot. *American Academy of Orthopedic Surgeons Symposium on the Foot and Ankle.* St. Louis, MO: CV Mosby; 1983:11.
15. American Academy of Orthopedic Surgery. *Orthopedic Knowledge Update: Home Study Syllabus.* 1984.
16. Insall JN, Falvo KA, Wise DW. Chondromalacia patellae: a prospective study. *J Bone Joint Surg.* 1976;58-A.
17. James SL, Bates BT, Osternig CR. Injuries to runners. *Amer J Sports Medicine.* 1978;6:40-50.
18. Olerud C, Rosenthal Y. Torsion-transmitting properties of the hindfoot. *Clin Orthop.* 1987;214:285.
19. Perry J. *Gait Analysis: Normal and Pathological Function.* Thorofare, NJ: SLACK Inc.
20. Coleman S. *Complex Foot Deformities in Children.* Philadelphia, PA: Lea & Febiger; 1983:7.
21. Bohannon R, Chauis D, Larkin P, Lieber C, Riddick L. Effectiveness of repeated prolonged loading for increasing flexion in knees demonstrating postoperative stiffness. *Physical Therapy.* 1985;64:494-496.
22. Hettinga D. Normal joint structures and their reaction to injury. *J Orthop Sports Phys Ther.* 1979;1:83-88.
23. Light K, Nuzik S, Personius W, Barstrom A. Low-load prolonged stretch vs. high-load brief stretch in treating knee contractures. *Physical Therapy.* 1984;64:330-333.
24. Catlin MJ, Dressendorfer RH. Effect of shoe weight on the energy cost of running. *Med Sci Sports Exerc.* 1979;11:80.
25. Frederick EC. The energy cost of load carriage on the feet during running. In: Winter DA, Norman RW, Wells RP, et al, eds. *Biomechanics IX-B.* Champaign, IL: Human Kinetics Publishers; 1985:295-300.
26. Frederick EC. Kinematically mediated effects of sports shoe design: a review. *J Sports Sci.* 1986;4:169-184.
27. Frederick EC, Howley ET, Powers SK. Lower O_2 cost while running in air cushioned type shoes. *Med Sci Sports Exerc.* 1980;12:81-82.
28. Nigg BM. *Biomechanics of Running.* Champaign, IL: Human Kinetics Publishers; 1986.
29. Nigg BM, Morlock M. The influence of lateral heel flare of running shoes on pronation and impact forces. *Med Sci Sports Exerc.* 1987;19:294-302.
30. Jorgensen U. Body load in heel-strike running: the effect of a firm heel counter. *Amer J Sports Medicine.* 1990;19(2):177.
31. Foster BK. Claw toes. In: Evarts CM, ed. *Surgery of the Musculoskeletal System.* New York, NY: Churchill Livingstone; 1983:9-153.
32. Sproul J, Hobart K, Mannarino F. Surgical treatment of Freiberg's infraction in athletes. *Amer J Sports Medicine.* 1993;21(3):381.
33. Rodeo SA, O'Brien S, Warren RF, Barnes R, Wickiewicz TL, Dillingham MF. Turf toe: an analysis of metatarso-phalangeal joint sprains in professional football players. *Amer J Sports Medicine.* 1990;18(3):280.

34. Harrington T, Dracr KJC, Dip RACOG, Anderson IF. Overuse ballet injury of the base of the second metatarsal: a diagnostic problem. *Amer J Sports Medicine.* 1993;21(4):591.

35. Baer GJ. Fractures with chronic arthritis. *Ann Rheum Dis.* 1984;2:269-273.

36. Devas MB. Stress fractures. *Practitioner.* 1966;197:70-76.

37. Ha KI, Hahn SH, Chung M, Yang BK, Yi SR. A clinical study of stress fractures in sports activities. *Orthopedics.* 1991;14(10):1089.

38. Marshall P, Hamilton WG. Cuboid subluxation in ballet dancers. *Amer J Sports Medicine.* 1992;20(2):169-175.

39. Pfeffinger LL, Mann RA. Sesamoid and accessory bones. In: Mann RA, ed. *Surgery of the Foot.* 5th ed. St. Louis, MO: CV Mosby; 1986:223.

40. Tanz SS. Heel pain. *Clin Orthop.* 1963;28:169.

41. Kibler WB, Facsm CG, Chandler TJ. Functional biomechanical deficits in running athletes with plantar fasciitis. *Amer J Sports Medicine.* 1991;19(1):66-71.

42. Holt KWG, Cross MJ. Isolated rupture of the flexor hallucis longus tendon. *Amer J Sports Medicine.* 1990;18(6):645.

43. Henry AK. *Extensile Exposure.* 2nd ed. New York, NY: Churchill Livingstone.

44. Johnson RE, Kirby K, Lieberman JS. Lateral plantar nerve entrapment: foot pain in a power lifter. *Amer J Sports Medicine.* 1992;20(5):619.

45. Jackson DL, Haglund B. Tarsal tunnel syndrome in athletes: case reports and literature review. *Amer J Sports Medicine.* 1991;19(1):61-65.

46. Radin EL. Tarsal tunnel syndrome. *Clin Orthop.* 1983;181:167-170.

47. Ferkel RD, Karzel RP, Del Pizzo W, Friedman MJ, Fischer SP. Arthroscopic treatment of anterolateral impingement of the ankle. *Amer J Sports Medicine.* 1991;19(5):440.

48. Boytim MJ, Fischer DA, Neumann L. Syndesmotic ankle sprains. *Amer J Sports Medicine.* 1991;19(3).

49. Ray RB, Coughlin ES. Osteochondritis dissecans of the talus. *J Bone Joint Surg.* 1947;29:697-706.

50. Canale ST, Belding RH. Osteochondral lesions of the talus. *J Bone Joint Surg.* 1980;62A:97-102.

51. Schwellnus MP, Jordan G, Noakes TD. Prevention of common overuse injuries by the use of shock absorbing insoles. *Amer J Sports Medicine.* 1990;18(6):636.

52. Jernick S, Heifitz NM. An investigation into the relationship of foot pronation to chondromalacia patellae. In: Rinaldi RR, Sabia ML, eds. *Sports Medicine.* Mt. Kisco, NY: Futura Publishing; 1979:1-31.

53. Eng JJ, Pierrynowski MR. Evaluation of soft foot orthotics in the treatment of patellofemoral pain syndrome. *Physical Therapy.* 1993;73(2):62-67.

54. Keating EM, Faris PM, Ritter MA, Kane J. Use of lateral heel and sole wedges in the treatment of medial osteoarthritis of the knee. *Orthopedic Review.* 1993;22(8):921.

55. Sasaki T, Yasuda K. Clinical evaluation of the treatment of osteoarthritic knees using a newly designed wedged insole. *Clin Orthop.* 1987;221:181-187.

56. Tohyama H, Yasuda K, Kaneda K. Treatment of osteoarthritis of the knee with heel wedges. *International Orthopedics.* 1991;15:31-33.

57. Yasuda K, Sasaki T. The mechanics of treatment of the osteoarthritic knee with a wedged insole. *Clin Orthop.* 1987;215:162-172.

58. Müller W. *The Knee: Form Function and Ligament Reconstruction.* New York, NY: Springer-Verlag; 1983:195.

59. Green WT. Discrepancy in leg length of lower extremities. *American Academy of Orthopedic Surgery Instructional Course Lecture.* St. Louis, MO: JW Edwards; 1951.

60. Dugas R, D'Ambrosia RD. Causes and treatment of common overuse injuries in runners. *Journal of Musculoskeletal Medicine.* May 1991:68.